Reclaim Your VOICE

Jaime Vendera

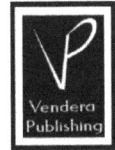

Copyright © 2013 by Jaime Vendera/Vendera Publishing

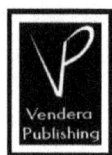

All rights reserved. No part of this book may be reproduced in any form, by any means, electronic or otherwise, including photocopying, scanning, downloading, or by any data storage system, without written permission from the publisher.

Interior Design: Daniel Middleton
www.scribefreelance.com

Cover Design: Molly Burnside
www.crosssidedesigns.com

Editor: Richard Dalglish

ISBN: 978-1-936307-30-2

Printed in the United States of America

CONTENTS

INTRODUCTION 5

Voice RX 7

    STEP 1: HYDRATE 9

    STEP 2: ELIMINATE 12

    STEP 3: MINIMIZE 16

    STEP 4: VOCALIZE 17

    FOR SINGERS ONLY 20

    BONUS: HOW TO BEAT A COLD 22

Vocal RESET 25

    REST 28

    ELIMINATION 33

    OVER-THE-COUNTER DRUGS 36

    SMOKING 36

    SUPPLEMENTATION 38

    ELEVATION 39

    TONING 41

    SEVEN-DAY PROGRAM REVIEW 43

    THE 5 & 10% RULE 44

The Air & Water Diet 49

    DRINKING MORE AIR 52

    EATING MORE WATER 58

LIVING THE AIR & WATER DIET	61
PROGRAM REVIEW	64

PractiSing 69

PROCRASTINATION ELIMINATION	71
VOCAL SELF-EVALUATION	80
PRACTISING APPLICATION	83

INTRODUCTION

Since 1996, I've taught countless singers the simplistic steps to maintaining their voices night after night on the road, and while in the studio. I've spent countless hours along the way perfecting each step to assure minimal time and maximum effectiveness. My methods have been described through books like *Raise Your Voice 1 & 2, The Ultimate Breathing Workout,* and *Sing Out Loud*, as well as mini-booklets such as *Voice RX*. After countless emails and texts from singers (including singer Myles Kennedy from Alter Bridge and Slash) praising my methods and sharing stories of how they've kept my books in their gig bags while on tour, and wishing that my booklets (*Voice RX,* etc.) were in print as well, I've finally decided to compile a quadrology of my booklets for keeping the voice in top shape. Thus was born *Reclaim Your Voice,* the compilation of *Voice RX, Vocal RESET, The Air & Water Diet,* and *PractiSing*. I hope you enjoy this compilation, keep it in your gig bag, and use it wisely when the need arises.

Jaime Vendera

Voice RX

Welcome to *Voice RX*. If you bought this book, chances are you're struggling with a sore throat. Struggle no more, because I've found the solution! My name is Jaime Vendera, and I am a professional vocal coach. I use my voice every day for hours on end. Since my voice is my job, without it I would be unemployed. I love my job, so I knew I couldn't let this happen. One of my specialties is working with touring singers worldwide, helping them recover lost voices. Touring and gigging singers come to me when they have lost their voice and want me to help save them from canceling that night's show because of a cold or vocal abuse on the road. By giving them some guidance, I've had singers singing entire shows without anyone knowing they couldn't speak an hour before, and I've even had the pleasure of helping rock stars sing night after night while battling a cold or the flu. Over the years, I developed a simple system that I give to every singer on the road. As a result, they are well prepared for any sore throat situation, even without my assistance. Thus *Voice RX* was born.

Voice RX isn't just for singers; it's for everyone who communicates. I know how important it is to have your voice in peak performance condition regardless of how you use it. Most of us use our voices daily, whether we're singers, speakers, phone operators, telemarketers, radio announcers, auctioneers, office workers, contractors, preachers, factory workers, schoolteachers—just about everyone except Blue Man Group and Silent Bob. It's our voices that do most of the communication, and when we lose our voice, we can feel lost. Feel lost no more, for there is hope! If you've lost your voice because of a cold or some other circumstance, you can still recover it to a level that will allow you to continue communicating.

If you've lost your voice and are struggling to regain it, *Voice RX* can help! Whether you have a sore throat from a cold, your throat feels extremely dried out, or your sinuses are clogged from a sinus infection or extreme hot or cold temperatures, you can regain your voice. Even if your voice is completely gone after a long night of performing, rehearsing, holding forth at a loud party, shouting at a ballgame, or having too much fun (can one have too much fun?), you CAN regain your voice! To repeat: if you've ever woken up with a sore throat, this program is for you. What I am about to reveal is not rocket surgery (yes, I meant to say rocket surgery). This is a systematic approach that I developed to help singers recover from a hoarse, sore voice to prepare them for their next gig, when time is a crucial element. I've had emails from performers telling me about times they had to sing the night after destroying their voice the night before, but once they used *Voice RX*, they could sing like a bird.

Voice RX looks at the whole range of voice users—singers, speakers, and general communicators—and presents the best and quickest fix to restore a "shot" voice. It's based on my personal experiences battling the same issues and my development of vocal techniques that have produced positive results for hundreds of singers.

Before going on, I'd like to state that I am not a doctor or vocal health specialist, and the following program is not intended to treat, prevent, or diagnose any general health or vocal health issues that may be related to your specific situation. This program has produced positive results for my own voice, but I urge you to consult your physician before trying any steps in this method. I am in no way responsible for the outcome or results you achieve through this process.

Let's jump right in and skip the boring explanations. I'll break it down into four simple steps. If you wake up with a sore throat, and you know it's most likely from singing all night, shouting at a game, partying a little too hard, or sleeping under a fan, then you need to Hydrate, Eliminate, Minimize, and Vocalize. Are you ready to try these four steps with me? Good, then let's get started.

STEP 1: HYDRATE

When you wake up with a sore throat, your voice is most likely in desperate need of water. Your vocal cords are probably dehydrated and swollen from misuse and abuse, and you'll need to get as much water into your system as possible to lubricate them. When the cords are low on water, the mucus that coats and protects them becomes thick, gooey, and yellow, which will hamper their ability to vibrate properly. To properly protect the cords and keep them well conditioned, the mucus coating them should be thin, clear, and watery.

Think of mucus as your engine oil. It keeps the cords "well oiled" and prevents them from overheating and swelling. You should change your car's engine oil every 3,000 miles, or it could become thick and dirty and possibly damage the engine. You have to change your voice's "oil" every single hour of every single day, or the oil that coats your cords will become sluggish, thick, or nonexistent, leaving the cords to overheat and burn out.

Getting the cords back to their well-oiled condition requires a three-step hydration process. This isn't quite as simple as just drinking water, because it will take approximately twenty minutes before the cords receive any benefit from a drink of water. Your cords are always the last part of the body to benefit, because the body's water reserve is dispersed in order of importance, and organs such as the kidneys and liver rank much higher than the cords on the scale of importance. Here are the three steps to hydrating and lubricating your voice:

1. Drink Water- When you first wake up, drink at least twenty ounces of water. That's not much. I bet many of you wake up and down a bottle of Mountain Dew. If you can do the Dew, you can do the water! Remember, it takes at least twenty minutes before you feel the effects of water on your cords. If you're spitting up thick, yellow phlegm, it's a good sign you aren't getting enough water. If you continually have sore throats in the morning, this could be one of the reasons. A good rule of thumb is to drink a half ounce of water per pound of body weight per day. If you weigh two hundred pounds, you need one hundred ounces of water every day. If you aren't meeting your daily requirements, begin immediately and you WILL notice improvements in your voice. Drink water throughout the day, not all at once. You need to change your "oil" every hour! For purposes of *Voice RX*, twenty ounces first thing in the morning gets the voice recovery process started.

2. Breathe Steam- By breathing steam, you immediately moisten the lungs, sinuses, and vocal cords. More moisture equals happy nose, lungs, and throat. There are several different ways to breathe steam. You can use a portable facial steamer, such as the Vicks Facial Steamer; you could hang your head over a sink with a faucet running hot water and breathe the steam while covering your head with a towel (the towel helps trap the steam); or you can take a hot shower. When you're on the road, you could turn the shower on in your hotel room and let the room fill with steam, or you can use a humidifier. I use a portable steamer for at night, (one that accommodates a 20-ounce water bottle) when I'm traveling for a glass-breaking show or vocal seminar, and I also run the shower in my hotel room for about thirty minutes, turning my room into a steam room before the performance. Okay, thirty minutes is a lot, but I tend to be a bit extreme. Steaming with any of the above methods for five to ten minutes will suffice for most people.

Before moving on, I'll mention that this program is also about maintaining a healthy voice. You now know that you should drink plenty of water every day, but you should also consider steaming every night. At home, run a steamer in your bedroom while you sleep. This not only hydrates the cords but also keeps your sinuses in good shape. You can use a hot or cold steamer or humidifier, whatever works for you, but please clean it every two to three days by scrubbing the interior with warm water and peroxide. Bacteria can build up in your steamer, and you don't want to breathe spores when sleeping (or any other time). If the walls inside your steamer are coated with a brown slimy substance, then it needs a good cleaning! I use a Venta-Sonic steamer at home, which has both hot and cold steaming options, as well as a water filter.

3. Mist Inhaling- I stumbled across this years ago, and I mean YEARS ago. When I was seventeen, I had a very bad case of strep throat. To ease my suffering, I was using a popular over-the-counter (OTC) throat spray every ten minutes. (Note: Now that I know about the alcohol content, I would never recommend using an OTC spray.) One time when I started to spray it in my mouth to relieve my throat pain, for some mysterious reason I start inhaling as I was spraying. It made me cough and gag, and I was very uncomfortable for a few minutes, but then suddenly I was pain free. I had actually breathed the mist down my trachea (the tube to the vocal cords and lungs), thus coating and numbing my cords. After I recovered from strep throat, I went to a local drugstore and bought a one-ounce spray bottle. I filled it with distilled water and tried a little experiment with mist inhaling. Inhaling water mist worked so well that I began inhaling all the time, especially when practicing, rehearsing, or performing. Mist inhaling allows a person to breathe in small water particles all the way down to the cords and lightly coat them, a simple trick to add "oil" to your voice.

Not to get sidetracked, but I'll mention that there are some great voice sprays on the market, like Throat Saver by superiorvocalhealth.com, and Vocal Eze by travelwellness.com, which many people use religiously. I don't begrudge singers and speakers using a good spray, but I strongly recommend not using it continuously. I use both Throat Saver and Vocal Eze, but I wouldn't squirt it down my throat between each song or every five minutes. Think of a spray as "food for voice." Sprays are something to aid in the vocal health process but shouldn't be your saving grace. Nothing works better for mist inhaling like plain, clean water! And remember, not all sprays are created equally. Stick to something like Throat Saver and Vocal Eze or do some research to make sure your chosen spray won't dry you out.

With that said, I suggest you adopt this third hydrating tip as part of your daily vocal regime. You should now be mist inhaling throughout this entire process.

STEP 2: ELIMINATE

In this step, our goal is to eliminate any bacteria that might be hanging around in the mouth, nose, or throat that could be causing a sore throat. Stressing and straining the vocal cords by shouting or over-singing can allow bacteria to sneak into the weak area overnight. So can drinking alcohol. But we also must realize that we are faced with airborne bacteria daily. By minimizing bacteria, we keep the voice strong and healthy. Whenever you're fighting a cold, or the voice is stressed, overworked, or dehydrated, or you go to bed without practicing oral hygiene (you know, brushing, flossing, gargling), you're setting up a possible home for bacteria to breed. So eliminate and your voice will feel great! There are three steps in the elimination process.

1. **Oral Hygiene-** Brush your teeth several times daily to get rid of bacteria, and scrape your tongue with a tongue scraper. You'd be surprised at the amount of bacteria that grows on your tongue overnight. Then rinse your mouth with some type of mouthwash. Although there are several ways to get rid of bacteria in the mouth, the method I use does not involve the use of any alcohol-based mouthwash. I begin by rinsing my mouth with plain water. Then I use hydrogen peroxide as a gargle. This kills bacteria without the drying effect of an alcohol-based mouthwash. If you don't like using peroxide, you can find several brands of alcohol-free/antiseptic-free mouthwash online or from a local health food store. Same goes for toothpaste and toothbrushes. Many people are anti-fluoride, so find a toothbrush and toothpaste that suit your needs.

   I use a mixture of baking soda and sea salt as my tooth cleaner and a Cybersonic toothbrush in place of a regular toothbrush (hey, I was in one of their commercials!). The Cybersonic has an interchangeable tongue scraper, flossing attachment, and toothbrush head. After one minute using the Cybersonic, my mouth feels minty clean, and my teeth feel as if they had just been cleaned at the dentist. Don't believe me? Check out my smile in one of my videos on YouTube, ha-ha. If you want a Cybersonic, or you want to learn more about it, go to sonictoothbrush.com.

2. **Sinus Irrigation-** The next step in the elimination process is sinus irrigation. Believe it or not, the sinuses should be cleaned every day, just like brushing your teeth. Even Dr. Oz agreed with me on this point when I appeared on his show. We inhale pollutants every day, which spread bacteria through the sinuses. Luckily, our sinuses are filled with cilia, which are the little hairs that try to catch those airborne irritants, thus keeping them away from our throat and lungs. However, those irritants are still lodged in the sinuses, and if

not eliminated can cause problems such as postnasal drip, stuffy and clogged nostrils, and sinus infections, which can all lead to a sore throat and cold.

The best way to eliminate these irritants is by using a Neti pot. "What's a Neti pot?" you ask. It's a little hand-held pot that looks like a genie's lamp, and it's used to flush water through the sinuses. I first learned about Neti pots in 1993, when I was addicted to sinus inhalers. I knew the inhalers were only making matters worse, because I had developed recurrent congestion. Recurrent congestion is when your sinuses react to the inhaler as an irritant and try to flush it from your sinuses. Every time I'd use the inhaler, I'd breathe fine for several minutes, but then my sinuses would become stopped soon after those few minutes of relief. Why? Because my sinuses were trying to naturally flush the spray from my nasal cavity, and the only way for the body to flush the sinuses is by producing more mucus. The mucus continued to build up heavily in my nose, and a vicious cycle was born that led to serious sinus infections.

I knew there had to be a better way, so I researched natural methods for clearing the sinuses. I read a book on yoga and found the answer in the Neti pot. Once I began flushing my sinuses, I was able to throw away my over-the-counter inhalers, and I have not used any since!

If you're addicted to an inhaler, throw it away immediately, head to a local store, and pick up a NeilMed NasaFlo Neti pot. It's the best Neti pot on the market! By now you should be wondering, "How do I use a Neti pot?" I'm glad you asked. You simply remove the top lid, add a mixture of warm water and salt, screw the lid back on and then stick the spout into one nostril, tilt your head and let the water flow out the other nostril. When you're finished, repeat the process through the other nostril. Sounds gross, doesn't it? Or maybe you think I'm trying to get you to water-board yourself. Trust me, it's not that bad, and you will be amazed at how much better you can breathe. If you can't find a NeilMed Neti pot, go directly to neilmed.com. There you'll see other sinus irrigation products, including a SinusRinse kit, which allows a little more irrigation pressure, and an electric irrigation system, which allows for serious sinus clearing. All kits come with prepackaged pharmaceutical-grade salt, which is very important, because your typical iodized table salt can irritate the sinuses. If you need salt this instant, get a container of non-iodized sea salt for best results.

As you flush each nostril with one full Neti pot, don't be alarmed if thick yellow mucus or little brown chunks come out. (Yes, I know, I know, but if you want to help yourself, you'll just have to get over the yuck factor.) The sea salt breaks up the stagnant mucus and dried blood, and the water pressure flushes the mucus and blood out of the sinuses, freeing the sinus cavity of obstacles, restoring balance and freedom for the cilia to do their job, and removing a home for bacteria to breed. If you're still a bit confused about sinus flushing, NeilMed has demonstration videos on their website for all of their products. Bottom line: flush your sinuses! I just found out a rock star friend of mine had postnasal drip for years. He bought a Neti pot, flushed his sinuses twice, and for the first time in years, found a solution to his problem. Sinus flushing works.

3. The Ultimate Gargle- The last step in the elimination process is to gargle the following solution: Mix one cup of hot distilled water, preferably boiled (microwaving adds harmful radiation to the water), with one tablespoon of organic apple cider vinegar, ¼ teaspoon of non-iodized sea salt, ¼ teaspoon of cayenne pepper, and five to ten drops of organic lemon juice. Once mixed, let the solution cool. Gargle this solution three to five times. Make sure it's not so hot that it burns your throat. I'll break down the benefits of this solution.

The water is a neutral solution to lubricate the mouth and pharynx. Hot water is best for relaxing the tissue in the throat, and, believe it or not, helps to reduce inflammation. Cold water will shock the vocal cords. (Imagine if someone dumped a five-gallon bucket of cold water on top of your head. Your whole body would tense up in shock. By the time you recovered, the perpetrator would be long gone.) When you drink ice-cold water, you do the same to the muscles surrounding the pharynx and vocal cords, which are right beside the esophagus (the tube that leads to the stomach), so the entire area feels the shock of cold water.

Apple cider vinegar (ACV) kills bacteria. It's important to note that if you buy a bottle of ACV from any old store, it won't work. It MUST be ORGANIC ACV! Why? It hasn't been filtered to take out all the nutrients that are important to vocal health. I suggest visiting a health food store or going online and purchasing a bottle of Bragg's Organic Apple Cider Vinegar. Bragg's ACV has not been processed or filtered. It still contains all the important nutrients for killing bacteria. These nutrients have been eliminated from the brands available at your local grocery store. You'll notice that Braggs is cloudy and not transparent like other brands. This is where ACV gets its potency, because all the nutrients reside in the cloudy part. So don't be alarmed if it looks like a fresh algae bloom or a large typhoid colony—it's okay if it's cloudy; in fact, if it's clear, it's no good for our purpose.

Salt is a natural cleanser because it breaks up mucus. Yes, I know it has a drying affect, but we've already got this part covered with the first step of this series. If you use sea salt, it won't feel as drying to the voice and will work to break loose and help flush mucus. I hate to repeat myself, but my suggestion is that you purchase organic sea salt. Iodized salt can be vocally irritating and doesn't work nearly as well.

Instead of using a dash of red pepper from the cupboard, I use two capsules of cayenne pepper. I open up the capsules, which contain about ¼ teaspoon, and add to the solution. You can get a bottle of cayenne capsules from any local health food store.

Cayenne pepper helps increase blood flow to the throat. You can use regular red pepper, and I even know of singers who use Tabasco sauce. The main purpose is to increase the circulation of blood to the voice so that it can quickly heal itself and naturally reduce the swelling.

Lemon juice has been used for years as a method of vocal relief. Truth is, lemon juice actually aggravates the cords because of its acidic nature. However, a few drops of lemon juice is an excellent way to get the glands salivating and help bring moisture to the mouth, which is a blessing on those mornings when you wake up with cotton-mouth. It's best to use organic lemons or lemon juice, if possible.

The purpose of this solution is to kill bacteria, break up mucus, increase the blood flow to the voice, and get the juices flowing (or get the glands producing saliva). Onto the next step.

STEP 3: MINIMIZE

You must minimize the amount of swelling of the cords in order to get them back into working order. You're probably asking, "If we want to reduce vocal cord swelling, why are we trying to get the blood flowing to the cords?" The answer is, because they are swollen from abuse and only by bringing the blood flow back into the cords will we be able to naturally reduce the swelling and make the vocal cords pliable again. When hoarse, the cords are rigid. Pliability is the answer. The key to reducing swelling is to feed the voice one zinc tablet and two capsules of licorice, followed by massaging the front of the throat. This relieves vocal tension, gets blood flowing to the cords, and starts the healing process. You can purchase zinc lozenges and licorice capsules online or at any health food store. Check out vitacost.com for the best brands and pricing. (You can even buy liquid versions of each from vitacost.com if you don't like taking pills.)

Why zinc and licorice root? Zinc is THE singer's mineral. It helps to rebuild vocal tissue. When choosing a zinc lozenge, make sure to bypass zinc gluconate lozenges—they're the ones that look and taste like candy. Most zinc gluconate tablets contain glycerin, which coats the pharynx, but if coating the throat is one of your goals, the better choice is slippery elm root, which is a natural demulcent. Slippery elm can be found in teas like Throat Coat Tea, by Traditional Medicinals, and lozenges such as Thayers Slippery Elm Lozenges.

Zinc gluconate tablets also contain sugar, which isn't good for the voice, because white sugar zaps our vocal energy. You'll end up eating them like candy, when the goal is to allow the tablet to dissolve in the mouth. When allowed to dissolve in the mouth, zinc will enter the bloodstream through the taste buds, which speeds up their potency for vocal recovery. Find a solid 23 mg zinc tablet that has a chalky feel and taste, and allow it to dissolve in your mouth. If you can't stand the thought of sucking on a chalky tablet, Liquimins liquid ionic zinc is the next best thing. I purchase mine from vitacost.com

Licorice is a form of natural cortisone, which helps to reduce swelling. When you're hoarse, it's a sign that the cords are swollen. Licorice will lessen the swelling.

Now let's massage the throat: Gently grab, squeeze, and release the skin on the front of the throat, starting at the bottom and working your way up to the chin. You can massage your throat as long as you feel it is necessary. This may be only five minutes or up to an hour. Your goal is to release tension in the throat area, however long it takes. If you want a more thorough breakdown of a massage routine for the voice, check out the Vocal Stress Release program from my book *Raise Your Voice Second Edition*. Once the muscles in the throat begin to relax, it's time to finish this system by doing some vocal warm-ups. Now it's time for the last step.

STEP 4: VOCALIZE

I have two vocal coaches who taught me amazing techniques for recovering a lost voice. My vocal coach Elizabeth Sabine, who taught singers from bands such as Guns N' Roses, Stryper, Megadeth, and 38 Special, told me that the vocal fry sound can be used to internally massage the cords and reduce swelling and is extremely valuable when you have a hoarse voice. Vocal fry is that sound you make when you wake up in the morning. You stretch and make a very low, kind of gritty, almost "non-tonal" sound. It reminds me of an old door slowly creaking open. This is actually the slow vibrations of the vocal cords touching and releasing as air passes between them on the lowest note you can produce.

The key to using vocal fry to recover your voice is to use it in moderation. When you wake up, right before, during, or after your water intake, do five to ten vocal fry sounds. Take a deep breath and go "ahhhhhhhhhhhhh" on a fry. Keep the volume and pitch very low and relaxed. It shouldn't take much energy to do a vocal fry, and if done properly, it will massage, not irritate, the vocal cords. Focus on feeling the sound "rumble" up in the roof of your mouth (the palate). The vocal fry brings energy and focus back into the throat. It tells the brain, "I need some help down here, can you send some blood flow and ease my pain?" For anyone who wants to know more about this sound, my *Raise Your Voice Second Edition* comes with audio examples that demonstrate vocal fry techniques.

My vocal coach Jim Gillette, who sang for the '80s metal band Nitro, taught me the best exercise I've ever known. Long before Jim taught me to shatter glass with my voice, he turned me on to an exercise called Lip Bubbles. Jim said Lip Bubbles (also known as motorboats, lip rolls, the baby buzz, etc.) were by far the best warm-up exercise on the planet. Lip Bubbles could not only warm up the voice for an amazing show but also help a singer recover a lost voice. When all else fails, and you think the show cannot go on, Lip Bubbles can save the day! Lip Bubbles WILL save the day and help you make it through your performance, do your speaking gig, talk on the telephone, and teach your class all day long.

Here's how to do this amazing exercise: after you've done five to ten vocal fry exercises, put your lips together ("purse" your lips) and begin to blow. This is the same vibrating sound a horse makes when it purses its lips and blows, making its lips flap loosely together. Channel your inner Mister Ed and try it a few times for fun.

Okay, fun is over, time for the work. Begin adding some sound to your voice as you flap your lips together. Your goal is to sustain a pitch while the lips "bubble" together. If you're having a bit of bubble trouble, you can lightly place your hands on each side of your face. This prevents the cheeks from puffing out, or filling up like a balloon, and concentrates the air right through the middle of the lips. Another tip is to pretend that you are going to say the word "bubble" as opposed to another word, like "pebble." Many singers try to start Lip Bubbles with a "P," when the exercise should start with a "B."

The reason Lip Bubbles are so beneficial is because once the lips "bubble," you've created two vibrating sources, your vocal cords and your lips. This cuts the vibrating source equally in half between the two. This means that you've lightened the load on the vocal cords, allowing them to rebuild and regain strength at a moderate rate. Think of it as physical therapy for the voice.

Lip Bubbles get the vocal cords to function properly by touching and releasing along the edges of the cords at every spot. When you abuse the cords, they swell and lose their ability to touch at every spot, which means you won't be able to hit certain pitches until you reverse the swelling. Swelling prevents the cords from touching and releasing as they normally do. Our goal is to gently work the cords together and get them touching at each spot for each pitch. Lip Bubbles are as close to massaging the vocal cords as you can get (except maybe for gargling water, which you might want to try). Bubbles are the best exercise I know for getting the blood flowing to the cords in record time.

Lip Bubbles sound like "bbbbbb" and should always begin with the consonant "B." When you make this sound, keep it as bubbly and soft as possible. You never want to do this exercise loudly or breathily, because excessive breath or forced volume aggravates the cords, and we are aiming for the opposite. Keep your Lip Bubbles light in volume and clean sounding (non-breathy).

To begin getting the blood flowing back into the area of the vocal cords and relieving the hoarseness, simply do ten to twenty Lip Bubbles on random pitches. Hold each pitch for a few seconds, and then slide to the bottom of your range. With each Lip Bubble, your voice will begin to open up and feel better. If you are really in a pickle and having trouble with your voice, you can do Lip Bubbles as long as you need, even throughout the day. I always use Lip Bubbles whenever I do a glass-breaking show. As long as I do them, I can scream for hours. I do them before the show, in between shattering a glass, and afterwards to "cool down" my voice.

I also offer the *Voice RX Warm Up*, which is a series of vocal scales that can be performed in fifteen minutes. I even sing them right along with you. You can purchase the *Voice RX Warm Up* download at venderapublishing.com or theultimatevocalworkout.com. As I said, I'll perform each exercise with you. Just follow along with me on each exercise and your voice will feel better in no time. Remember to keep them light in volume, pure and clean in sound, and never strain for a note.

The *Voice RX Warm Up* exercises will cover one chromatic octave, in what I call the C to C system. You will hear three notes on the piano, covering three octaves, i.e., a low C, a middle C, and a high C. I designed it this way to incorporate everyone's range, for both male and female voices, allowing you to start wherever you feel most comfortable. If you get to the end of an exercise, and you need or want to work higher, just start the scale again and work as high as needed.

That completes the four-step program. I began using this method years ago and found that it also helped me to sing better when I was just plain physically drained. It helps reconnect the voice and will give you confidence that you CAN sing or speak in any situation. Using *Voice RX*, I've even performed on a glass-breaking show after lying in bed sick for six days. I got in front of the camera with a temperature of a hundred and two degrees, when only two hours before I couldn't even speak. How did I do? I shattered the glass! My wish is for *Voice RX* to work as well for you in any situation. With that said, it's time for you to apply the four steps in *Voice RX* so you can be on your way to vocal recovery. Good luck and keep me posted!

FOR SINGERS ONLY

If after the entire program, you are still hoarse or sore and need more of a workout to prepare your voice for a rehearsal or gig, etc., then you can use what I call the nine-song system. Basically, you are going to choose nine songs that you enjoy singing, three different songs for your low range, three different songs that work your midrange, and three songs toward the high end of your range. For example, if I was going to choose my first three songs, one of my picks for the low-range category might be *Bright Lights* by Matchbox 20. A choice for my midrange might be *Calling All Angels* by Train, or *Hallelujah* by Jeff Buckley, while one of my higher-range choices might be *Higher Place* by Journey, or the Police classic *Roxanne*.

After you have picked all nine songs, please put them into a CD or MP3 player in the following specific pattern from low to medium to high, three times in a row:

Low
Medium
High
Low
Medium
High
Low
Medium
High

After you have your playlist, use the following formula:

* Lip bubble the first three songs from low song first, then medium, then high.
* Hum three songs, low song first, then medium, then high.
* Sing the last three songs very softly and purely, almost so softly that you can't hear it, without whispering the song, as if a fly were singing them. Start on the low song, then the medium song, and finally the high song. If you aren't warmed up and vocally free of soreness, stress, and strain by the end of the nine-song session, then your problem could be the result of something else, such as acid reflux or laryngitis.

If you're experiencing symptoms of acid reflux, the magic cure is to take one tablespoon of Bragg's Organic ACV. Acid reflux is said to be caused by too much acid in the stomach, but some recent research suggests it's caused by too little acid in the stomach, which slows down the digestion process and results in food backing up the throat. Adding apple cider vinegar reestablishes the acid balance and will relieve symptoms of acid reflux in as little as five minutes. Acid reflux can also be dealt with by drinking Apple Cider Vinegar tea. Add a tablespoon of Bragg's Organic ACV and a tablespoon of pure honey to a cup of hot water and sip throughout the day.

If it is acid reflux, pay close attention to your diet. What seems to be causing the reflux? Is it your posture, or perhaps spicy foods or caffeine? Many foods and beverages can cause reflux. There are many resources on the Internet to help you play detective and solve your own case of the reflux dilemma, including my book *Raise Your Voice Second Edition*.

As well, a hoarse, tired voice that feels like acid reflux could be the result of sleep apnea. If you snore, wake up with a dry throat, and even more tired than before you went to bed, you're a candidate for sleep tests which must be ordered by your physician.

If your horse voice persists beyond several days, and you feel it may be more than tiredness, or reflux, and fear that you might have laryngitis, go to a doctor before your next show to find out for sure. If you have laryngitis, cancel your show. I strongly recommend you not perform with laryngitis. This is a time of vocal rest and complete vocal silence. Speaking of vocal silence, on days you use *Voice RX*, keep the talking to a minimum. Vocal fry and Lip Bubbles only, please!

Good luck, singers, I KNOW you will sound great tonight! I have faith in you.

BONUS: HOW TO BEAT A COLD

There are a kazillion things you could do for a cold, including going to the doctor, taking different herbs and vitamins, working up a sweat, old-time remedies, etc. But the following is what I do EVERY TIME I feel a little tingling in my throat, or I start to feel congested. Perform all four steps of *Voice RX*, but add the following to Step 2:

Vitamin C
Calcium/magnesium tablets
Colloidal silver

Take one vitamin C caplet, one calcium/magnesium tablet, and ten to fifteen drops of colloidal silver every hour until the tickle goes away. What's colloidal silver? Colloidal silver is small particles of silver suspended in water. Silver acts as an antibiotic, making it a highly effective bacteria and virus killer. Unlike other antibiotics, the body cannot develop a tolerance to it, making it very effective in stopping colds, flu-like symptoms, and sinus infections. I use it every time I feel any type of cold-like symptom coming on, and usually within a few hours I feel fine. It is important to note that vitamin C and calcium are some of the first nutrients in the body to be depleted under stress, which means stress just might be the cause of your cold or flu. So take a chill pill, relax, and don't stress so much.

When you start feeling sick, I'll bet you're low on these nutrients. I use calcium/magnesium tablets because magnesium helps the body absorb the calcium. (There is much debate nowadays on whether this is true, as there is with using colloidal silver, so do your own research and decide for yourself.) Calcium also helps to alkalize the body, and modern science tells us that infection cannot thrive in an alkalized environment; it breeds in an acidic environment. The body is either more acidic or more alkaline at any given time. Keep the body alkaline to stay healthy. I'm not an alkaline/acidic specialist, so please feel free to research this area as well. (I can tell you that former major league outfielder Al Kaline, who played 22 seasons with the Detroit Tigers, is in the Baseball Hall of Fame. Coincidence? I think not.) Among the things that make the body acidic are alcohol, caffeine, sugar, and stress. Things that alkalize the body include green leafy vegetables and calcium. Go alkaline!

If you don't like taking pills, I suggest using the water additives Emergen-C and X20 packets from singerswater.com instead. Emergen-C is a powder containing B vitamins, vitamin C, and trace minerals that you add to a bottle of water. You can buy it at any health food or grocery store. X20 is a sachet that contains coral calcium and trace minerals such as ionic zinc (it also helps to alkalize the body) that's added to your water. A packet of Emergen-C and a sachet of X20 can supercharge your water, boosting your immune system while eliminating pill swallowing! Remember, X20 can be purchased through singerswater.com.

Now that your water is supercharged, let's revisit the sinuses. If you're flushing the sinuses but still experiencing congestion in your lungs or sinuses on a regular basis, you can add two tablespoons of organic apple cider vinegar to a steamer and breathe in through your sinuses for ten minutes. This will help kill any bacteria still lurking about after irrigation and will keep infection from spreading.

To further open the sinuses and lungs, rinse out your steamer and add a half cup of water and some essential oils, such as thyme and clove oil, to the mix. Thyme and clove will open the sinuses and lungs without a drying effect. If you don't have a portable steamer, boil a pot of water on the stove and inhale from the boiling pot of water.

Afterwards, feel free to flush your sinuses with salt water. The solution should be barely salty to taste. If it's too salty, it will sting your sinuses. If you're using NeilMed prepackaged salt, you won't have to worry about this. Remember, if you use regular iodized salt when flushing your sinuses, you'll get a bit dried out in the larynx, and the cords may feel irritated, so I always recommend organic sea salt or NeilMed packages.

That finishes *Voice RX*. Let me leave you with one last bit of advice. After you have performed the four-step process, give your voice plenty of rest. You need time to heal, so vocal rest is a must. If you have to perform on a certain night, or your job entails speaking throughout the day, I totally understand that you don't have much time to rest. But keep your talking to a minimum throughout the day, and when you must speak, do so at a moderate volume, drink plenty of water, mist-inhale frequently, and repeat *Voice RX* before hitting the stage. If your hoarseness is a prolonging nuisance, I suggest check out the next book in this series, *Vocal RESET*. Regardless, I wish you a speedy recovery and healthy voice.

Vocal RESET

After writing *Voice RX,* I realized that there are specific situations when a singer or speaker may need more than a quick fix, because a hoarse voice might not specifically be the result of a night of yelling at a game, singing too loud, or talking above the crowd. A hoarse voice and heavy phlegm on the vocal cords might be the result of poor vocal habits a singer or speaker has developed over a period of time, habits that have ultimatelyweakenedthe quality of his or her voice. If this sounds like your situation, you may need more than a one-day *Voice RX* fix.

If you've been continuously clearing your throat for months, cannot get rid of the phlegm that hangs on your vocal cords like a sticky spider web, and have a nagging pain in your throat and recurring feelings of heartburn or sinus drainage, it might be time to "reset" your voice.

I created *Vocal RESET* to give singers and speakers the power to regain their voice. However, this program is NOT a quick fix or vocal bandage; it is simply a way to reinstall healthy vocal habits, eliminate bad vocal habits, and give your voice time to adjust to the new patterns.

> **WARNING:** This program is extreme and requires full commitment! Although it's simple, it may be too extreme for you to handle, depending upon your current condition. *Vocal RESET* was not designed to fix a broken voice; it was designed to help in the process of regaining what you've vocally lost. I am not a doctor or vocal health specialist, and the following program is not intended to treat, prevent, or diagnose any general health or vocal health issue that may be related to your specific condition. If you decide to try the *Vocal RESET* program, please consult your physician.

What is *Vocal RESET?* As the name implies, it's a simple way to "reset" your voice back to its basic nature, while discovering—and eliminating—the causes of vocal irritation and swelling. If you continue abusing your voice through poor technique, bad vocal habits, constant vocal abuse, or poor diet and then ignore the warning signs, those signs (sore throat, hoarseness, etc.) will eventually intensify. As time passes, it will become increasingly difficult to bring your voice back to a fully functional, healthy state. The result could be permanent vocal damage, such as nodules on the vocal cords. Yes, nodules can be removed by surgery and, if caught in time, can even be naturally reversed with vocal therapy, but why put yourself through that? If you clear your throat every day, if your voice always feels dry, if you feel you've lost range, or if your voice has felt brittle, tired, sore, or raspy for a long time, you're a prime candidate for *Vocal RESET.* Let's begin.

Vocal RESET is an acronym I dreamed up while driving one day (thank you, Lord). It's based on five principles that together will create a healthy "vocal environment" for regaining a healthy voice. *Vocal RESET* is a seven-day program that must be strictly followed.

Let me emphasize that "strictly followed" message: You can reset your voice in seven days if you follow the program precisely—no cheating. If you do, you'll be on your way to a better voice. It's a simple program but not necessarily an easy one, because it requires eliminating the things in your life that can negatively affect the voice, such as smoking and caffeine. Therefore, I also created what I call the *5&10% Rule*, which is a method that continues beyond the seven-day program. It's designed to slowly and easily wean the smoker and caffeine junkie off of Camels and Mountain Dew. (Remember: There are no old Camel smokers!) But first the basics; the basic seven-day program consists of the following:

RESET=

Rest

Elimination

Supplementation

Elevation

Toning

By applying all five elements—Rest, Elimination, Supplementation, Elevation, and Toning—you can "reset" your voice to project a pleasing tone; get rid of that husky, irritating rasp; give your voice the rest it needs for regaining vocal stamina; and regain confidence in the sound of your own voice. Heck, most of us have a problem enjoying the sound of our own voice even when we're vocally healthy. It must be nearly impossible to enjoy your voice when you're dealing with a continual sore throat or recurring rasp. But help is at hand. *Vocal RESET* will break down each factor of the acronym so that you fully understand how to apply each step in the seven-day program.

A note on the *5&10% Rule*. Singers or speakers who are heavy smokers, drinkers, caffeine junkies, etc., will want to add the *5&10% Rule* to the seven-day program, as described at the end of this book. I say that because I've been there myself; it took me thirty days to kick my caffeine habit. If you just nodded and smiled, you know what I'm talking about. But the *5&10% Rule* makes it easier to break bad habits and deal with moderate withdrawal symptoms at a controlled pace.

Before we start, please purchase a notepad or journal to keep notes throughout the seven-day program. It will be your *Vocal RESET* diary. Every day, you will take notes on all five factors so that we can "crack the code" on whatever is causing your vocal trouble. I want to help you to not only reset your voice but also become aware of how you got into vocal trouble in the first place. Anyone who has read my books should have guessed that I'd require you to do some writing. Everyone knows I *am* a diary nut. Even if you hate to write, you must keep a daily diary; it's critical to your ultimate success. Nuff talk, let's get started:

REST

Your voice is shot, devoid of power. It sounds wimpy and breathy, and you feel vocally drained. Sounds like you need some rest! Singers sometimes forget that they need to rest their instrument! You ARE your instrument, and if you don't give yourself adequate rest, the vocal tissue can't repair itself. Recite this mantra: "I am always healing, I am always healing, I am always healing ... "

It's true; you ARE always healing! If you cut your finger, the cut heals; if you get a cold, your immune system eventually defeats the virus that caused it; if you lose your voice, it eventually comes back. Healing is what God intended, BUT, for healing to take place, you MUST get the rest you need. If you do not get both adequate sleep and vocal rest, you will feel it in your voice!

When a singer constantly feels pain or an ache in their throat after speaking or singing, it could indicate a number of factors, not only lack of rest but also lack of water, dietary issues, and poor vocal technique. *Vocal RESET* will address all of them except vocal technique. If you want to learn more about vocal technique (which, as a singer, you should), check out my book *Raise Your Voice Second Edition*.

Regardless of your technique, once your voice is shot, you need rest. Rest heals the body and voice; it recharges your batteries. The first part of *Vocal RESET* will address recharging your batteries through both sleep and vocal rest. Let's start with sleep:

SLEEP

It's time for some self-analysis. How much sleep do you get each night? Five hours? Seven hours? Ten hours? Do you wake up refreshed or feeling more tired than when you went to bed? Believe it or not, getting too little OR too much sleep can equally affect your body, making you tired and groggy. If you wake up feeling more tired than when you went to bed, it's a safe bet that you need some sleep adjustments. If you feel refreshed in the morning, then you can skip this section and keep doing what you're doing. Jump ahead to the Vocal Rest section. But if you're sleep deprived, read on.

We're going to test your sleep patterns to discover whether or not you're getting an adequate amount of sleep for your body. So I'll ask again: How many hours do you sleep per night? Answer this question accurately. You'll need to know the correct answer in order to proceed. Grab your journal or notepad and write a heading for a section called "REST." Below that heading, write down the amount of sleep you typically get every night. I also want to know how you feel in the morning when you wake up.

Let's say you sleep eight hours per night. If you feel refreshed in the morning, remember, there's no need to adjust your amount of sleep, just skip ahead to the Vocal

Reclaim Your Voice

Rest section. But if you do not feel refreshed when you wake up in the morning, you'll need to write down how you feel. Do you feel grouchy? (Write down "feel grouchy" in your journal.) Does it take you twenty minutes to pull yourself out of bed? (Write down "took 20 minutes to get out of bed" in your journal.) Does it feel like it takes several hours just to get your speaking voice back? All of this information is very important. *You must write everything down in your journal.* Don't procrastinate, or you might forget. Jot down the information when it's fresh in your mind. It's one less thing to do later.

Don't worry about making your notes sound as if Shakespeare wrote them, and don't worry about spelling, grammar, and punctuation (I'm trying to make this as easy as possible so that you'll do it, that's how important it is.) Just jot down your thoughts. For example: *I feel more tired when I wake up than when I go to bed … I wake up all through the night … My voice is froggy every morning … I wake up and can't get back to sleep … I wake up in the middle of the night and see extraterrestrial aliens standing next to my bed watching me.*

Our sleep cycles occur in 90-minute intervals, and if you're suddenly awakened during a 90-minute sleep cycle, it could affect how refreshed you feel. If you wake up several times through the night, you may be affecting the cycles, and it could be one reason you sleep poorly.

If you're a sound sleeper and don't wake up in the middle of the night, but you're still tired in the morning, maybe you're disrupting a sleep cycle when you awake. If a sleep cycle lasts 90 minutes, it makes sense that a person should sleep in 90-minute chunks. Otherwise, their sleep patterns would be thrown out of whack, no? Wouldn't 7.5 hours (five 90-minute sleep cycles) serve a person better than eight hours?

With that said, please note that this is just my personal observation. I am not a sleep expert, and this book does not address the stages of sleep, such as deep sleep or REM sleep. The physiology of sleep is a complex subject better addressed in other books. If you want to learn about sleep cycles, there is an abundance of information on the Internet and in bookstores.

Since you're typically an "eight-hour" sleeper, the first step to discovering the amount of sleep you need is to try less sleep per night by adjusting to the closest sleep cycle below eight hours. Assuming 90-minute cycles, a new sleep cycle occurs at seven and a half hours. Set your alarm to get up thirty minutes earlier than usual. The next morning, when you've fully awakened, note any differences in your energy and mood. Do you feel better? Are you happier? Do you feel more refreshed? Make a new heading underneath the "REST" section in your journal for "DAY ONE" and list anything that comes to mind concerning how you feel that morning! Your journal is very important! (I might have mentioned that already.) It will probably take several days before you can truly answer these questions, so in keeping with the seven-day *Vocal RESET* program, try this "shorter" sleep pattern for the first three days, writing a new section in your journal for each day. Now, let's move on to the next experiment.

On the fourth day of the program, readjust your sleep time to allow a cycle beyond your typical eight hours. For the "eight-hour" sleeper, this extra sleep cycle would result in a total of nine hours of sleep (six 90-minute cycles). So, on the fourth night of this program you MUST get nine hours of sleep. Set your clock for an hour later than your usual "eight-hour" wakeup time. If this doesn't fit your work schedule, be prepared to go to bed one hour earlier. It may be tough adjusting to that extra hour, but you'll get used to it. Try this new pattern for three days. How do you feel? Refreshed, happier, recovered? Write it down in your journal. Continue this new pattern for three nights, making sure to write in your journal every morning. And don't forget to write in your journal.

On Day Seven of the program, review your sleep journal, which I know you've been keeping diligently. Which of the three sleep patterns work best for you? The usualamount of sleep?Less sleep? More sleep? There is no right answer; it depends on how you feel. By the seventh day, you should adapt to your new sleep pattern, using the notes in your journal as your guide.

You say you didn't notice a difference because you toss and turn throughout the night, and now you're wondering what to do? It's time to play sleep detective.

Do you snore? Ask your mate. No mate, no problem. Turn on a digital recorder tonight, listen tomorrow, and find out. If you are a snorer, it would be wise to consult your physician for a sleep test and follow the doctor's guidance. In the meantime, you could try snore strips to open your sinus passages. To keep your sinuses and throat moist through the night, run a humidifier during your sleep time. There are various "snore sprays" on the market that might help. I personally had better luck by simply filling a one-ounce misting bottle with distilled water and spraying it into the back of my throat before going to sleep. Snoring could also be caused by buildup in the sinuses. If you have sinus problems such as a stuffy nose, begin flushing your sinuses with a neti pot, as described in my books *Raise Your Voice Second Edition* and *Voice RX*. All of these tips can help eliminate snoring, so give them all a try and don't forget to check with your physician.

Supplements may help take you into the Land of Nod, including chamomile, kava kava, melatonin, and valerian root, among others. Do some research and decide if any of these will suit your needs. A word of caution: As a singer and speaker, I don't recommend using over-the-counter "PM" type sleeping aids, because they have a tendency to dry out the voice.

Another way to help induce sleep is visualization. One great way to slip into a deeper sleep state is by counting backwards from seven to one, while associating each number with a color, such as Red 7, Orange 6, Yellow 5, Green 4, Blue 3, Indigo 2 and Violet 1.

Visualize these actual numbers in your mind as if they are painted in each associated color. If you fully visualize each colored number thoroughly, you'll probably drift off to sleep before you finish counting. (If you don't like the colored numbers idea—or you find it difficult to keep track of which colors go with which numbers—you could count sheep, but that's old school. You might try counting free-range chickens or grass-fed buffaloes instead.)

VOCAL REST

Now that we've covered physical rest, it's time for vocal rest. This might seem a bit too strict for you to handle, but to reset your voice you MUST do it as I say in this book. Vocal rest is always tough for me because I can't keep my mouth shut for more than ten minutes, but if your voice is shot, you need a minimum of twenty-four hours of complete silence to begin the healing process. If you work, take a day off or take your vocal rest on the weekend. Ignore the telephone unless you believe there's an emergency. If a call is not about an emergency, let the caller know right away that you can't talk because you're giving your voice a rest and that you'll have time to gossip—oops, I mean chat—later in the week. If you have an answering machine, listen as the caller leaves a message before picking up the phone. You might even change your answering-machine greeting to something like, "Hi, this is Jaime. I can't talk right now because I'm giving my voice a much-needed rest. Please leave a message, and I'll get back to you Monday evening." (Don't forget to change your greeting back to the regular one after your voice rest.)

On the second day you can begin using the telephone if needed, but for no more than a few minutes at a time. Set a four-minute egg timer (or any other timer, like the one on your microwave) and end the call when the alarm sounds. Conduct all conversations in the same fashion. On Day Three you can begin talking more on the phone, up to ten minutes at a time. I'll even let you talk a bit more in person (Thanks, Jaime!), but keep it short. Avoid all unnecessary conversation. Every day after, you can add back a little more speaking until you reach Day Seven, when you can speak normally again. Take this time to realize exactly how much time you spend talking. Is all that chatter really necessary? Hey, I'm just asking, one chatterbox to another. I honestly don't care how much talking you do every day as long as you have some solid vocal technique under your belt. Vocal technique is just as important to speaking as it is to singing. When resetting your voice, learn to limit your conversations for a few weeks to give your voice the rest it needs. Giving a hoarse voice rest makes it happy.

Yes, I know most people use their voice for their job. You might need to schedule some days off for a "vocal vacation." What better way to rebuild your voice than to take an actual vacation? So head to the beach and relax. Take a book and read. But remember, no talking means no talking. Follow these guidelines to a "T" in order to reap the rewards.

ELIMINATION

All right, you've made it to the next part of *Vocal RESET*. Now it's time for some elimination, and to begin factoring out what might be causing your vocal irritation. A host of foods can trigger irritation, including dairy products such as milk and cheese and acidic foods like tomatoes and lemons. Substances such as alcohol and caffeine also can irritate the voice. During your seven-day program you MUST eliminate certain foods from your system and monitor any differences in your voice. I am teaching you to become your own vocal detective to figure out if any of your dietary choices are negatively affecting your voice.

Here is a checklist of seven basic vocal aggravators:

- Acidic and spicy foods (tomatoes, lemons, orange juice, etc.)
- Alcohol
- Caffeine
- Carbonated beverages
- Dairy products
- Over-the-counter drugs
- Smoking (of any kind)

The list above contains the most-common aggravators of the voice. If you use any of them, cut them completely out of your routine for seven days. There are many more foods, beverages, and substances that can affect the voice, and different people will react to different foods. If you're suspicious of anything in your daily regimen or diet, eliminate it as well. Now, before reading on, take out your diary and add a new heading titled "ELIMINATION." Write down the names of any foods, drinks, or other substances that you plan to cut out for the week. Let's look at each vocal aggravator in detail:

ACIDIC FOODS
Acidic foods can cause acid reflux, which will give you that throat burn or heartburn after you eat. Take a moment to reflect on your daily eating habits. Everything you eat or drink affects your body, whether for good or ill. If you notice that you eat lots of pizza and wake up with a sore throat, it could be because of the spiciness or acidity of the sauce. (It could also be the cheese, which we'll get to shortly). Eliminate any spicy or acidic foods from your diet for seven days.

If you gorge yourself when you eat (you know who you are), you might experience heartburn even if you didn't consume a jar of salsa or bucket of Buffalo wings. ("So,

Jaime, if I might get heartburn anyway, there's no point cutting out spicy foods, right?" "WRONG!") Gorging can also pack on the pounds. One way to avoid gorging is to eat more slowly. To eat more slowly, take smaller bites and chew your food well; proper chewing not only slows you down but also aids digestion. Instead of inhaling your lunch, take some time to actually taste it and enjoy it. Try chewing a minimum of ten times before swallowing (though a few more chews won't hurt you).

Another important rule to follow during the elimination portion of *Vocal RESET* is to eat your last meal at least three hours before going to bed. This gives your body time to digest your food. A good rule of thumb is no eating after seven o'clock. Why is this important? Because you don't want your body trying to digest food when you're also trying to sleep, which would interrupt the rest part of *Vocal RESET*. We want the body focused on repairing itself during sleep, not digesting those four huge slices of bacon pizza you hogged down during the ten o'clock news.

So, for seven days, please eliminate any spicy chicken wings, hot peppers, salsa, lasagna, orange juice, oranges, grapefruits, lemons—basically anything acidic or spicy—and do not eat within three hours of going to sleep. Write in your journal after every meal. Note how you feel physically and vocally every time you eat. Does your voice feel any better, or do you still notice negative signs? If phlegm is still building, or your throat becomes sore after eating, note which foods you're still eating. It might not be that morning jolt of grapefruit juice or that arrabbiata sauce you like to drown your penne in. It might be—anything! ANY food might be affecting your voice, which is why you need to undertake this process of elimination. It could take weeks, so I urge you to write everything in your journal until you figure out any and all foods that seem to negatively affect your voice.

After seven days you may begin eating spicy or acidic foods again, but I want you to pay close attention to how your voice feels after you eat these foods. In other words, continue writing in your journal after you reintroduce these foods to your diet. How do you feel physically and vocally after eating a bowl of chili or some curried chicken? Does your voice feel phlegmy, hoarse, or itchy? Remember, although spicy foods typically are the culprits, ANY food can affect your voice. Many people have a "food intolerance," and some have food allergies, although food allergies are much rarer. In the back of your journal, under the title "INTOLERANCES," keep a list of the foods that seem to affect you, and try to limit their consumption.

> **Note:** If eating spicy hot wings affects your voice, but you just can't live without them, you can help tame the flames by immediately drinking one tablespoon of organic apple cider vinegar (I prefer Bragg's) after scarfing the wings. (I

explain the benefits of apple cider vinegar in my book *Raise Your Voice Second Edition.*)

ALCOHOL

Alcohol will dry you out, plain and simple. Apply a little rubbing alcohol to your hand and watch it rapidly evaporate. This is what you do to your voice every time you take a drink. I pray you don't drink, but if you do, put it away for a week and see how your voice feels after seven days. If you enjoy beer or wine or something stronger, and you feel as if you can't give it up, I've created the 5&10% Rule, which you'll find at the back of the book. It describes a process to help wean yourself from that cold, frosty beverage.

CAFFEINE

Caffeineis a diuretic, which means it'll make you pee like an Arabian stallion. You will literally lose more water than you take in from that soda. If you're caffeine sensitive, as I am, it will make you feel as if you have a cobweb of phlegm on your throat that you just cannot get rid of no matter how loud and hard you hack up. (Sorry.) This is because that diuretic is pulling the moisture right out of your voice and leaving that mucus to coat the cords without being diluted by water.

"Ooh, mucus on the vocal cords, that's nasty." Listen up: We all have mucus on our vocal cords; it's thin, clear, and watery, and it protects the cords from becoming irritated and swollen. But that mucus needs to be diluted with a supply of fresh H_2O, or else it becomes thick and yellowish and clings to the cords like Velcro. Think of vocal cord mucus as new motor oil. If you don't "change your oil" by drinking plenty of water daily, that mucus will turn into sludge, like ten-year-old motor oil that's never been changed. Caffeine creates sludge, so put down the soda cup and the coffee mug for seven days. If you're a caffeine junky, add the *5&10% Rule* to the seven-day program.

CARBONATED BEVERAGES

Carbonation can cause acid reflux because the carbonation bubbles expand in the stomach, which can cause stomach acid to back up the esophagus. That's why you sometimes feel stuffed after drinking a carbonated beverage. If your beverage is bubbly, put it down for the week. You might notice you feel less bloated, which by itself is a great improvement. Need something sweet to replace it? Try "Throat Coat Tea" by Traditional Medicinals. This is a sweet-tasting herbal tea made for singers and speakers that contains soothing herbs for the voice.

DAIRY
Dairy products are sludge creators, and they will cause mucus buildup on the vocal cords, which makes it hard to speak and sing without hocking up a lougie. (Sorry.) Have you ever felt that way when drinking milk or eating a grilled cheese sandwich? If so, note it in your diary. While you're on this program, hide the milk and cheese please!

OVER-THE-COUNTER DRUGS
I am referring to cough medicines, sinus inhalers, cough drops, headache medicine, allergy relief pills, etc. All of these OTC medications can dry out your throat. Give them a break for a week. If you are a nasal mist junkie, keep track in your journal of how you feel. You might feel worse without your nasal inhaler or experience recurrent nasal stuffiness. Hang tough; you can do this program! If you feel like you won't make it without your OTC nasal inhaler or allergy pill fix, use a neti pot; it will help keep your sinus passages open.

SMOKING
Inhaling smoke of any kind destroys the voice! Smoke damages the little hairs, or cilia, that protect the sinuses and lungs. The tar you inhale coats your lungs. That's why heavy smokers have that "smoker's cough" all day long, you know, the one that sounds like they're trying to spit up a chunk of their lung. If you're a smoker, you'll definitely need to incorporate the 5&10% Rule, because you must wean yourself from smoking.

I am in no way an expert on smoking addiction, so I urge you to seek more support than this book offers. If you need further assistance, do what works best for you. I pray you eliminate smoking from your life. It's not only one of the worst things singers and speakers can do to their voices but also one of the worst things you can do to your body, period!

When eliminating smoke from your system, you might experience a "hacking up" similar to smoker's cough and think this program isn't working for you. Don't worry, that's the built-up tar in your lungs coming up and out. Stick with it. You've finally given your lungs the chance they've been waiting for to get rid of that tar. Your body is simply releasing nasty toxins, and you will feel better in the end!

Make sure to write down any symptoms you feel throughout the day. Do you have spurts of energy? Does your tone suddenly sound cleaner, or are you hacking up a lot? Are you jonesin' from lack of caffeine? Experiencing a headache? Do you feel tired at certain times during the day? These are simply side effects from caffeine withdrawal. You'll make it. Do you feel any better day-by-day? Do you feel less bloated since you quit drinking carbonated soda? It's very important to keep track of how you physically and vocally feel, especially after meals, so write everything down. Write everything down. Write everything down.

Reclaim Your Voice

After seven days, it's up to you to decide what to reintroduce into your diet and daily regimen. However, take note of how your voice feels. If you plan to reintroduce more than one substance or food, I suggest doing one at a time and waiting three days to reintroduce the next. If you're reintroducing three items, for example, it will take seven days, the first item on Day 1, the second on Day 4, and the third on Day 7. Meanwhile, pay attention to your body so that you can figure out which foods or other substances affect your voice the most, although I am sure they will all affect you in some manner.

For instance, if you love pizza and orange juice, reintroduce OJ for the first three days and then pizza afterwards. Keep notes in your diary as you add foods, OTC drugs, and beverages back into your daily routine. Did that OJ make your voice scratchy or make you feel as if the mucus was building up? Perhaps the sinuses got a little stuffy. Perhaps there wasn't any change at all. If there *were* definite negative side effects, remember to add them to your journal's "INTOLERANCES" list along with any foods, beverages, and substances that seem to affect your voice.

I am not trying to persuade you to quit drinking orange juice or adjust your lifestyle. I simply want to make you aware of what is affecting your voice and help you understand that the choices you make may be the problem. If you recognize the problem, you can begin formulating a solution.

SUPPLEMENTATION

If you've read my other books, most of this information won't be new to you, but there are certain supplements that feed the voice and immune system that every singer and speaker should take on a regular basis. So I've put together a short list of specific supplements I want you to take while on this program. This will be your "Voice Pack" of vitamins and minerals. If you want to know more about supplements, read *Raise Your Voice Second Edition* and *Superior Vocal Health*. Otherwise, head to the vitamin store and purchase the following:

- General multivitamin
- B-complex
- Calcium
- Vitamin C
- Zinc
- Licorice root
- Slippery elm

For every day of the seven-day program, take one multivitamin, one vitamin B complex, 500 mg of vitamin C, 1,000 mg of calcium, 23 mg of zinc, some licorice root, and some slippery elm.

Everyone needs a good multivitamin. Both vitamin C and calcium support the immune system. I want you to stay cold free as much as possible. After all, when we singers are sick, we seem to feel it mostly in our voice. It's better to boost the immune system and avoid the colds. Zinc is the singer's mineral and builds the vocal tissue. It's "food for voice." Slippery elm is a natural demulcent and will help make the lining of the throat feel slipperier. Licorice is natural cortisone and will help reduce some of that vocal swelling. Both licorice and slippery elm are in Throat Coat Tea. If you're drinking a cup a day, you've got these herbs covered.

If you prefer liquid formulas and want to boost your system with herbal combinations, check out the Superior Vocal Health line available through superiorvocalhealth.com.

ELEVATION

I would rather have used another word, but nothing else fit the RESET acronym, ha-ha. Basically, we need to "elevate" our hydration levels. In other words, it's time to drink up on water. Most people seriously underestimate the amount of water needed every day to keep not only the voice but also the entire body in smooth working condition. How much water do you drink every day? The norm is considered one half ounce of water per pound of body weight per day. If you weigh two hundred pounds, you'll need one hundred ounces of water throughout your day, every day. For this program we are going to waterlog your system using the following guidelines:

    Teens—One half gallon of water per day for seven days
    Women—Three quarters gallon per day for seven days
    Men—One gallon of water per day for seven days

This might seem extreme, especially if you aren't used to drinking much water, but it won't hurt you. Some people worry about water toxicity, but you would need to drink something like ten gallons of water in a day to harm your body, and the guidelines above require far less than that.

The water needs to be pure. Distilled water is best. So run out to the grocery store and buy seven gallons of distilled water and a fresh lemon. Squeeze the lemon juice into a one-ounce bottle that has a dropper top, or buy a dropper at the drugstore. Keep the juice refrigerated. Next, use a black marker to write a day of the week on each gallon container. When you crack open your gallon each day, add seven to ten drops of pure lemon juice to the water. Keep the drops small and add no more than ten; you shouldn't taste the lemon. The lemon juice will help your system absorb the water and flush your kidneys. You can also replace the minerals that are missing from distilled water by adding two X20 packets from singerswater.com to each gallon, which will super-charge your aqua!

If you're a teen or a woman and won't be drinking a full gallon per day, fill a two-liter bottle or a half-gallon jug with lemon-water each day, and drink till it's empty.

After seven days, adjust your water levels to the daily amount your body weight requires. The goal is to flush the body with a refreshing supply of water so that your system is well hydrated and the voice and sinuses have the H_2O they need to function properly. You'll notice that your voice feels better and wetter, and you produce sounds more easily. And it was that easy! If you don't like water, I don't know what to tell you. There is no alternative. NOTHING replaces water! So drink up and enjoy the benefits.

Don't forget to make notes in your diary. Check off each day as you reach your water quota. How does your voice feel from the extra water? Is your voice feeling more buoyant with every passing day? Is your voice feeling better as the seven-day program goes by? Write it all down, because it is very important to know!

TONING

Nope, I am not trying to turn you into a Buddhist monk. But by introducing toning into the program, you can begin finding your voice again. Reintroducing some pure, healthy vibration to your voice is therapeutic and relaxing. Toning should not come into play until the fifth day. Focus on four days of vocal rest first. Toning is easy; it's simply long, drawn-out humming.

To begin toning, lock your legs stiff and bend over until your hands and head hang toward the floor. Begin humming "mmmmmmmm" on any lower note in your speaking voice. Don't lock or hold your breath when doing this. Breathe from the belly as described in my vocal books. As you breathe freely and hum, you will feel the sensation of your voice "buzzing" your cheeks and nose. This is a good sign. You should always feel the buzzing sensation.

As you hum, open from "mmmm" to "aaaahhh," like "mmmmaaaahhh." The "h" should be silent, no breathiness. Stand up and try it again. You should not only feel as if the sound of your voice buzzes your entire face but also feel a buzzing in the roof of your mouth, like a zillion bees are tickling your soft palate. This is where you should feel the sensation of your voice at all times.

> **Note:** If your voice feels hoarse, consider trying this technique: buy a three-foot length of half-inch tubing like that used in aquariums. Put one end of the tubing into a tub of water and hum on the other end. The vibrations will carry down into the water and back up the tube, and your vocal cords will feel as if they are getting a vocal massage. It's a very therapeutic sensation and will help decrease the pain.

When speaking, if you feel the sensation of your voice fall down in your throat and become slightly throaty or raspy, you are using your voice incorrectly. Simply bend over and hum again to regain your buzzing tone. This "raspiness" is called "vocal fry." Vocal fry is that sound you have when you wake up in the morning and your voice is low and gritty sounding. If you're using vocal fry, you'll sound like Elmer Fudd from the Bugs Bunny cartoons. A little bit of vocal fry will help to massage the cords and warm them up, but a lot of fry will irritate them and cause swelling.

Don't confuse vocal fry with adding grit or screaming. That's a whole other ballgame and can be learned if you want to sing rock. I teach grit techniques at screaminglessons.com.

That sums up the seven-day program. Follow it and don't cheat! If you follow through, you will begin to understand your voice, and with understanding comes mastery. Master your voice; don't be a slave to it. Let's review:

SEVEN-DAY PROGRAM REVIEW

KEEP A DIARY
Write down any and all details concerning your voice during the seven-day program.

REST
Adjust your sleep patterns to 90-minute cycles, beginning with less sleep for the first three days, more sleep for the next three days, and adjusting to the best pattern on the seventh day. Begin the first twenty-four hours of the vocal rest process with complete vocal silence. Each day after, add more talk time.

ELIMINATION
Eliminate acidic and spicy foods (tomatoes, lemons, orange juice, etc.), alcohol, caffeine, carbonated beverages, dairy products, over-the-counter drugs, and smoking (of any kind) for seven days. Then it's your choice whether to pick up the old habits or not.

SUPPLEMENTATION
Begin your vocal pack of vitamins, which consists of a multivitamin, B-complex, calcium, vitamin C, zinc, slippery elm, and licorice. If you want more herbal combinations for the one-two punch, check out the Superior Vocal Health line at buildabettervoice.com.

ELEVATION
Drink up on water! Kids, a half gallon; women, three-quarters gallon; men, a full gallon, every day for seven days. After seven days, adjust your water intake to your body weight based on one-half ounce of water per pound of body weight per day.

TONING
On the fifth day of the program, bend over and hum "mmmmmmmaahhhh." Feel that sensation in your cheeks and nose. Stand up and maintain that buzz when you speak. Feel it in the roof of your mouth. Make sure to use correct vocal technique for breathing and vocal placement, as explained in *Raise Your Voice Second Edition*. If you lose the buzzing sensation and the voice gets gritty, bend over start humming again to find the buzz. Maintain the buzz.

That's all there is to *Vocal RESET*. Now, if you have a habit (such as smoking) that you cannot quite eliminate for seven days, the next section was created just for you.

THE 5 & 10% RULE

The *5&10% Rule* is for smokers, drinkers, caffeine addicts, sinus spray lovers, pizza freaks, and anyone else with a hard-to-break habit that may be affecting your voice. It's an extension of the seven-day program that may last anywhere from two to six weeks, depending on your consumption levels. If you're a moderate caffeine drinker, you can be free in a few weeks. If you're a heavy smoker, it could take thirty days or longer. The whole point of this program is to gently wean yourself away from anything you want to eliminate from your daily consumption.

Luckily, I am not addicted to any of these substances, but I do understand that some habits are tough to kick. So I only offer this advice as an additional support measure for kicking that habit. My advice may need to be supplemented by the help of a doctor or counselor as well as products developed to help combat withdrawal symptoms. When I weaned myself off of caffeine, I took aspirin to relieve the caffeine headache I experienced. I urge you to do some research on the side effects associated with your habit before following my suggestions.

Follow the seven-day program as noted above, but adjust the "Elimination" step as follows:

5% RULE

All you'll need to do to apply the *5% Rule* is cut your consumption by 5% every day, whether it's cigarettes, soft drinks, milk, or an occasional beer or cocktail. By eliminating 5% a day you can slowly rid your body of these aggravators, and you can be free and clear of your addiction usually within thirty days. When using the *5% Rule*, you do not continue to remove 5% of the original amount each day. Instead, you remove 5% of that day's amount, so the 5% gets smaller. I'll give you a full example so you can understand the power of this program.

Let's say you smoke two packs of cigarettes a day (forty cigarettes per day). Using the 5% rule, you will eliminate 5% of each day's amount, as follows:

Day 1 — 40 cigarettes minus 5% (2 cigarettes), leaves you with 38 cigarettes to smoke.

Day 2 — 38 cigarettes minus 5% (1.9 cigarettes), allows you 36.1 cigarettes. (Okay, I don't expect you to smoke .1% of a cigarette, so when using the 5% rule, always round up fractions of what you're eliminating to the next number. So 5% of 38 cigarettes = 1.9, which rounds up to 2 cigarettes, leaving you with 36 cigarettes to smoke on Day 2. Note that even 1.1 cigarettes would round up to 2.)

Day 3	– 36 cigarettes minus 5% = 34 cigarettes (eliminating 2 cigarettes)
Day 4	– 34 cigarettes minus 5% = 32 cigarettes (eliminating 2 cigarettes)
Day 5	– 32 cigarettes minus 5% = 30 cigarettes (eliminating 2 cigarettes)
Day 6	– 30 cigarettes minus 5% = 28 cigarettes (eliminating 2 cigarettes)
Day 7	– 28 cigarettes minus 5% = 26 cigarettes (eliminating 2 cigarettes)
Day 8	– 26 cigarettes minus 5% = 24 cigarettes (eliminating 2 cigarettes)
Day 9	– 24 cigarettes minus 5% = 22 cigarettes (eliminating 2 cigarettes)
Day 10	– 22 cigarettes minus 5% = 20 cigarettes (eliminating 2 cigarettes)
Day 11	– 20 cigarettes minus 5% = 19 cigarettes (eliminating 1 cigarette)
Day 12	– 19 cigarettes minus 5% = 18 cigarettes (eliminating 1 cigarette)
Day 13	– 18 cigarettes minus 5% = 17 cigarettes (eliminating 1 cigarette)
Day 14	– 17 cigarettes minus 5% = 16 cigarettes (eliminating 1 cigarette)
Day 15	– 16 cigarettes minus 5% = 15 cigarettes (eliminating 1 cigarette)
Day 16	– 15 cigarettes minus 5% = 14 cigarettes (eliminating 1 cigarette)
Day 17	– 14 cigarettes minus 5% = 13 cigarettes (eliminating 1 cigarette)
Day 18	– 13 cigarettes minus 5% = 12 cigarettes (eliminating 1 cigarette)
Day 19	– 12 cigarettes minus 5% = 11 cigarettes (eliminating 1 cigarette)
Day 20	– 11 cigarettes minus 5% = 10 cigarettes (eliminating 1 cigarette)
Day 21	– 10 cigarettes minus 5% = 9 cigarettes (eliminating 1 cigarette)
Day 22	– 9 cigarettes minus 5% = 8 cigarettes (eliminating 1 cigarette)
Day 23	– 8 cigarettes minus 5% = 7 cigarettes (eliminating 1 cigarette)
Day 24	– 7 cigarettes minus 5% = 6 cigarettes (eliminating 1 cigarette)
Day 25	– 6 cigarettes minus 5% = 5 cigarettes (eliminating 1 cigarette)
Day 26	– 5 cigarettes minus 5% = 4 cigarettes (eliminating 1 cigarette)
Day 27	– 4 cigarettes minus 5% = 3 cigarettes (eliminating 1 cigarette)
Day 28	– 3 cigarettes minus 5% = 2 cigarettes (eliminating 1 cigarette)
Day 29	– 2 cigarettes minus 5% = 1 cigarette (eliminating 1 cigarette)
Day 30	– NICOTINE FREE

10% RULE
All you need to do for the 10% Rule is cut your consumption by 10%. (You probably figured that out.) Let's say you're a caffeine junky and you drink a six-pack of Pepsi every day. If you applied the 5% Rule, it could take nearly seven weeks to completely wean yourself off of caffeine. The 10% Rule will speed up the process.

Jaime Vendera

Note: With cigarettes, we counted actual cigarettes, but with beverages, we'll count ounces as opposed to how many bottles of soda you drink. This means you'll need a few measuring utensils. It also means that some days you'll waste some of your drink. Whereas foods can be stored, soft drinks can't. It's best to pour the daily excess down the drain so you won't be tempted to finish it off.

In the following example, our caffeine junky drinks six twenty-ounce bottles of Pepsi per day, which equals 120 ounces of soda. Here's how to eliminate that caffeine addiction in record time:

Day 1 — 120 ounces minus 10% = 108 ounces (eliminating 12 ounces)
Day 2 — 108 ounces minus 10% = 97.2 ounces (eliminating 10.8 ounces)
(Again, you don't get to drink that extra .2 ounces, just as you couldn't smoke that .1% of a cigarette. Always round up, which means 10.8 ounces = 11 ounces, bringing your consumption on Day 2 to 97 ounces. All right, already one bottle down!)

Day 3 — 97 ounces minus 10% = 87 ounces (eliminating 10 ounces)
Day 4 — 87 ounces minus 10% = 78 ounces (eliminating 9 ounces)
Day 5 — 78 ounces minus 10% = 70 ounces (eliminating 8 ounces)
Day 6 — 70 ounces minus 10% = 63 ounces (eliminating 7 ounces)
Day 7 — 63 ounces minus 10% = 56 ounces (eliminating 7 ounces)
Day 8 — 56 ounces minus 10% = 50 ounces (eliminating 6 ounces)
Day 9 — 50 ounces minus 10% = 45 ounces (eliminating 5 ounces)
Day 10 — 45 ounces minus 10% = 40 ounces (eliminating 5 ounces)
Day 11 — 40 ounces minus 10% = 36 ounces (eliminating 4 ounces)
Day 12 — 36 ounces minus 10% = 32 ounces (eliminating 4 ounces)
Day 13 — 32 ounces minus 10% = 28 ounces (eliminating 4 ounces)
Day 14 — 28 ounces minus 10% = 25 ounces (eliminating 3 ounces)
Day 15 — 25 ounces minus 10% = 22 ounces (eliminating 3 ounces)
Day 16 — 22 ounces minus 10% = 19 ounces (eliminating 3 ounces)
Day 17 — 19 ounces minus 10% = 17 ounces (eliminating 2 ounces)
Day 18 — 17 ounces minus 10% = 15 ounces (eliminating 2 ounces)
Day 19 — 15 ounces minus 10% = 13 ounces (eliminating 2 ounces)
Day 20 — 13 ounces minus 10% = 11 ounces (eliminating 2 ounces)
Day 21 — 11 ounces minus 10% = 9 ounces (eliminating 2 ounces)
Day 22 — 9 ounces minus 10% = 8 ounces (eliminating 1 ounce)

Reclaim Your Voice

Day 23 — 8 ounces minus 10% = 7 ounces (eliminating 1 ounce)
Day 24 — 7 ounces minus 10% = 6 ounces (eliminating 1 ounce)
Day 25 — 6 ounces minus 10% = 5 ounces (eliminating 1 ounce)
Day 26 — 5 ounces minus 10% = 4 ounces (eliminating 1 ounce)
Day 27 — 4 ounces minus 10% = 3 ounces (eliminating 1 ounce)
Day 28 — 3 ounces minus 10% = 2 ounces (eliminating 1 ounce)
Day 29 — 2 ounces minus 10% = 1 ounce (eliminating 1 ounce)
Day 30 — 1 ounce minus 10% = 0 ounce (eliminating 1 ounce)

Wow, it's kind of funny how both examples worked out to be nicotine and caffeine free on the same day. That was just a coincidence. Whatever you want to eliminate, simply figure out your daily intake, grab a calculator, and do some calculations to see whether 5% or 10% works best for you.

This ends the *Vocal RESET* program. If you want to regain your voice, this is a great way to start. I hope you've enjoyed this program, and I truly hope it helped. See you next book.

The Air & Water Diet

Welcome to the *Air & Water Diet*. If you're tired of riding up and down on the lose-weight/gain-it-back elevator, and if you yearn for the energy you had when you were twenty, reading this booklet can be a step in the right direction. But, before we begin, I must state that this is NOT an actual diet. The *Air & Water Diet* is a new way of life or, better yet, a return to a natural way of life, one you were born to live. By returning to the natural, correct way of breathing, and by meeting your body's hydration requirements with good old water, you CAN and WILL increase your metabolism, which will give you a more desirable body weight while increasing overall health and energy.

What is metabolism and what does it have to do with our weight? Metabolism is the rate at which your body uses oxygen to burn the fuels we ingest into our body (i.e., food), which in turn feeds the body, strengthening the organs, muscles, and tissues. The more oxygen we consume, the more efficiently we burn our fuel; the more efficiently we burn our fuel, the less fat we'll pack onto our cells. Plainly put, metabolism turns fuel into energy and new cells.

If you follow this super-simple program, it will stoke your internal fat-burning flames, help flush your system of unwanted toxins, and give you a new burst of raw, natural energy, without downing an energy drink.

For those worried about breakfast, lunch, and dinner, don't worry, this isn't some weird starvation diet where you'll be living on air and water in an attempt to shed excess pounds. We're not going to replace your eggs, soups, snacks, and steaks with a big bowl of oxygen. You're simply going to discover an easy way to increase your air and water intake to aid the digestion of the foods you love. So you can breathe easy (no pun intended), because you do NOT have to quit eating what you are eating now, although adjusting your food choices and the amounts you consume may help. Let me repeat: This is not some fad food diet approach to counting calories and adjusting carbs, and I won't promise that you'll drop 18 pounds in four days.

Here's more good news—this program does not require you to perform an hour of grueling exercise every day in order to shed a pound of pure fat per week. (But I have included a super-simple exercise section to encourage a bit of sweating.) Nor is this a program to flatten your tummy, tone your tush, or build your biceps (but don't be surprised if you notice a difference in body tone). This is a simple, easy-to-remember program for the majority of us who are wiped out from a full day of work, who would love to slip in some exercise, and who wish they had the willpower to diet but are too tired, too unmotivated, too weak, or just too lazy to incorporate any sort of routine.

The *Air & Water Diet* is based on the scientific fact that increasing oxygen and water intake WILL increase and improve metabolism. Unfortunately, as a society, our metabolisms have plummeted because of physical and mental stress from work and life in general as well as poor eating habits. Years of consuming pounds of junk food, gallons of caffeine, and mountains of white sugar, salt, and flour have taken a toll on many of us.

Through stress and horrible eating habits, we've watched our metabolism leap out of our bodies and run for the door, while we sat crying, our faces buried in a hot fudge sundae as our energy melted away like the whipped cream on top. I'm not a nutritionist, far from it. I'm not a personal trainer or a diet consultant. Yet in my career as a vocal coach, I've heard complaints about weight and energy time and time again. I've listened to people—performers who felt they lacked enough stage stamina to perform at the top of their game night after night—beg for solutions. I've seen them slouching, trying to suck in their gut while chomping on a fast-food hamburger chased down by a slurp of soda, wondering where their energy went.

What I noticed in these cases is a deficiency of water intake and incorrect breathing habits. Sadly, these shortcomings are typical for many singers, including those skinny, wound-for-sound ones. Many people who lack energy (my singers included) suffer because of scant water intake and faulty breathing habits, often indicated by their short-windedness. People have forgotten how to breathe. They've become shallow breathers, proudly puffing out their chests and sucking in their guts, which, while it might make them look like newly minted Marines, unfortunately limits their oxygen intake. They've turned to soft drinks as their main source of hydration, and they munch on chips for a quick energy fix. Junk food lacks the air and water present in raw foods such as apples, and we now understand that insufficient intake of air and water plays havoc with our bodies, throwing our metabolism out of whack, which can result in weight gain, bad skin, fatigue, poor overall health, and a poor vocal performance for all you singers reading this. These dire consequences can lead to further complications and spark a downward spiral.

We've turned into a caffeine society driven by coffee, cola, energy drinks, and five-hour energy fixes as our only source of hydration and rejuvenation. We've replaced water with caffeinated substitutes that actually rob the body of hydration! That's because caffeine is a diuretic that'll make you pee your brains out as it destroys your skin cells and wreaks havoc on your adrenal glands and overall system. Meanwhile, the sugar in your coffee and soft drinks give you a temporary energy rush that does more harm than good. Have you ever noticed how an hour after you've eaten a candy bar, drunk a soda, or downed an energy drink, you're ready to crash and go to sleep? That's because the sugar in those junk foods increases the amount of insulin in the bloodstream, which boosts energy. But to avoid too much insulin, the body rapidly decreases blood glucose, which leaves you tired. We are slowly destroying our bodies and taking years off our lives because we've developed poor eating, breathing, and drinking habits. It's time to regain control.

So, why did I write this book? I wrote it because I realized that what I was doing as a vocal coach to help improve a singer's voice was also improving their health. But I also wrote it to address my own health issues. My main gig as a vocal coach and glass-shattering celebrity keeps me hopping. I personally struggle with health issues that cause me discomfort when traveling the world performing on television shows. I finally grew tired of struggling with my energy levels and turning to prednisone to keep me in balance, so I woke up one day and thought to myself, "Jaime, you preach diet, exercise, water, and breathing to all your students, yet you ignore your own advice. Do something about it!"

I finally did something about it during the summer of 2012, when my health again declined. I watched my weight rise and fall like a yo-yo. I quit exercising, choosing instead to take naps several times a day. I felt as if I had chronic fatigue syndrome, yet I ignored it. Then one day, the solution unfolded before me. If I couldn't get up and exercise, I'd figure out a method to substitute for it, a sort of "couch potato cardio," if you will. The *Air & Water Diet* is the result.

Believe it or not, the genesis of this book was a bunch of forgotten notes I'd written as a continuation of my book *Vocal RESET*, the final installment of my *Voice RX* trilogy, which helps singers struggling with vocal problems. It has since morphed into much more, but it still serves the same purpose. Over the years, because of my own physical allergies, I've had to adjust my way of life. Singers must stay healthy to maintain a great voice. Besides doing vocal exercises and singing, singers must take into consideration their food choices, water intake, breathing, and, of course, exercise. All four factors affect the voice. With that said, I've put together a super-simple kick-starter program based around all four (air, water, and yeah, a little bit of diet and exercise) that will work for anyone (not just singers) who wants to take back control of their metabolism and regain the energy of their youth. Let's get started.

> **DISCLAIMER:** The following sections are not intended to prescribe, treat, prevent, or diagnose any illness. Consult your physician before attempting any of the following exercises or testing any listed products, vitamins, minerals, or herbs.

DRINKING MORE AIR

There are tons of diet books and workout programs on the market; this book is NOT one of them. I want to present you with a nearly FREE way to improve your health and reap the benefits almost immediately. Let's begin with air, because air is free (although keeping it clean—or at least nontoxic—is not free). Walk outside and take a big gulp of clean air. If you live in a smog-laden city, take a trip, find a forest, hug a pine tree, and breathe, breathe, breathe. Feels good, doesn't it? Breathing is easy, we already know how to do it, and most of us are active enough to do it every day—there's something about that staying alive thing that motivates us. Now it's time to go beyond typical breathing. It's time for some real breathing!

WHY AIR?

If breathing is so easy that it's automatic, why dwell on it? Because air is important not only for living but also for living with quality. Air is our fuel. It feeds the cells. For singers (and anyone who opens his or her mouth and expects words to pour out), it's the fuel that vibrates our vocal cords to create our tone. For one hundred percent of the population—singer, speaker, and cloistered monk alike—it's also what stokes our fat-burning furnaces. Air primes the metabolism and stokes those tiny little fires in each of our cells, helping them burn hotter, thus burning more fat cells. This isn't a scientific explanation, but hey, did you buy this book for a science lesson or to change your life? I figured as much, so I'll keep the explanations on my level (third-grade, in case you were wondering). To get you excited, here are some of the benefits of deep, natural breathing and drawing more oxygen into the body:

- Detoxifies and releases toxins
- Releases muscular tension
- Calms and clears the mind
- Relieves pain
- Massages the organs
- Strengthens the immune system
- Helps remove carbon dioxide from the blood
- Strengthens the lungs and heart
- Promotes cellular regeneration

- Improves mood
- INCREASES ENERGY LEVELS VIA IMPROVED METABOLISM
- AIDS DIGESTION

YES, I meant to spell the last two in ALL CAPS because that's exactly what this book is about! Do you want more energy? Do you want to lose those unwanted pounds? Do you want to improve your health, live longer, calm your mind, get rid of muscle pains? Then proper breathing is part of the road to recovery!

Oxygen does the body good. Countless studies have revealed the benefits of cardiovascular exercise, proving that increased oxygen = increased metabolism = increased energy = increased fat-cell burning. If you're gaining fat, I'm betting you're taking in more junk than oxygen. Plain and simple, cells either release energy or form fat. With more fat, a cell can process food with less oxygen, but it just keeps building and building. Before long, those size 2 jeans from high school magically transform into size 22, until one day you look at yourself in the mirror and say, "How did *that* happen?"

This is why my singers, especially the ones who follow the program from my book *The Ultimate Breathing Workout*, tell me they have much more energy, have lost weight, and feel much better overall. Oxygen feeds your internal fire! When you increase your oxygen, you speed up your metabolism and increase your body's ability to stimulate enzymes that burn fat.

Here's what happens when you deprive your body of oxygen (and it's worse than just weight gain): You starve your cells, thus your engine is not functioning at maximum capacity. In addition, you accumulate toxins and garbage, affect digestion, prevent the body from absorbing the proper nutrients, decrease metabolism, continue to gain fat, feel more tired and sluggish, have poor-looking skin, and age faster.

Increasing oxygen availability results in a number of benefits. More oxygen increases the intestines' ability to process nutrients, and this change can begin to occur within a matter of minutes.

To dispose of fat already stored within the body, it must be combined with oxygen to burn it. Research has shown that a large percentage of Americans use less than 25 percent of their lungs' capacity. Merely increasing oxygen intake through proper breathing can increase the body's ability to burn fat by 100 percent or more.

The process by which the body loses weight and creates energy depends on a substance called adenosine triphosphate (ATP). Oxygenating body cells through effective breathing produces an environment that encourages production of this substance.

Cortisol and insulin are also produced within the body. Normally these chemicals are beneficial, but stress can prompt their overproduction over extended periods of time. This leads to many destructive effects, one of which is the storage of fat. Proper breathing keeps the bloodstream oxygenated, reduces stress, and decreases cortisol production.

Another major function of the body is the removal of toxins. Modern-day invaders such as food preservatives can decrease the effectiveness of the glands that regulate weight. Even worse, the body can form more fat in an effort to store those toxins. Well over half of these toxins can be converted into gases that can be expelled from the body. Studies by one California clinic indicated that proper breathing technique could increase removal of these toxins by more than 10 percent.

If you breathe more efficiently and take in more oxygen, you'll also feel better emotionally. That's because you'll send a signal to the brain to release endorphins, that feel-good bodily drug. You've probably heard about the phenomenon known as the "runner's high." If you've ever run a marathon, half-marathon, or even a five-mile race, you were undoubtedly breathing efficiently. If not, you probably found yourself standing on the side of the road, clutching your sides, wheezing, and watching the other runners go by. The runner's high comes from all that air, and you can experience the feeling while sitting on the couch, instead of running for an hour on the treadmill.

That click you just heard was the light bulb switching on inside your head. Yes, this is the lazy man's way to exercise. By the end of this book, you'll be performing "couch potato cardio" like a pro!

So, where did your breathinggo wrong ? Or did it go wrong? Was it ever right? I'm sure you once had excellent breathing habits, but breathing is so obvious that we can take it for granted and get off track. We can jump back on by taking the following correct-breath test to learn if we're breathing right:

1. Stand in front of a mirror.
2. Inhale as deeply and quickly as possible, while watching yourself in the mirror.
3. Exhale as deeply and quickly as possible while watching yourself in the mirror.
4. Repeat until you are sick of taking this test.

Time for test results. Did you:

A. Suck in your stomach as you inhaled?
B. Puff out your chest as you inhaled?
C. Raise your shoulder as you inhaled?
D. Puff out your belly as you inhaled?

Which one are you? Don't worry about the exhalation for now. If you didn't get the inhalation correct, that exhalation won't matter. There's only one correct answer: D. If you sucked in your stomach, puffed out your chest, lifted your shoulders, or did all three, you're committing respiratory suicide. Your belly should look like an inflating balloon as you suck in all that air, otherwise you're way off track.

What, my lungs are down in my stomach?

No, no, no, don't flip out on me. Your belly only appears to be filling with air because you are utilizing correct breathing, that is, *diaphragmatic* breathing. The diaphragm is a muscle that rests along the bottom edges of the ribs. Its purpose is to contract to create a vacuum in the lungs so the lungs can easily draw in air. But because the lungs are basically air sacks, we can fill them without using the diaphragm. As a result, many of us have forgotten the natural way of breathing, allowing A, B and C (sucking in the stomach, puffing out the chest, and raising the shoulders during inhalation) to wreak havoc on our breathing machine.

There's one group that does know how to breathe properly, and we can learn from them. The members of that group are ... babies!

Watch a baby lying in its crib. Notice how his little belly rises and falls. That is correct breathing. Most of us think that when we inhale, we're supposed to suck in our gut and puff out our chest while raising the shoulders. WRONG! That's society's mistake. In fact, it should be completely opposite. Sucking in the gut fights against the diaphragm, impeding efficient inhalation. When we breathe, the diaphragm should drop down, effortlessly contracting, which will cause our back, side ribs and belly to protrude, or expand outward. That's because the diaphragm presses down on the lower organs, forcing them outward and opening up the lungs via a vacuum. As a result, the lungs can completely fill, flooding our bodies with oxygen.

Imagine a crackling fire in an old stone fireplace. The logs are burning nicely, smoke is rising through the open chimney, and you can feel the air near the fireplace gently wafting toward the flames as the fire draws the oxygen it needs to burn. Now imagine closing the flue and closing the glass doors in front of the fireplace. The fire will die from lack of oxygen, and theroom will fill with smoke (the hearthside equivalent of the toxins the body needs to rid itself of). When we suck in the gut, puff out the chest, or lift the shoulders on an inhalation, we're smothering the body's fire, so it won't burn efficiently. We leave old, stagnant air trapped in the lungs because we're barely filling them up; we've shut the furnace doors. Exhalation is one way we release toxins, so if we fall into a shallow breathing pattern, we suffer two ways—we limit fuel supply on the inhalation and toxin release on the exhalation.

Take a lesson from the babies. Watch them again. See their little bellies rise on the inhalation while their shoulders stay relaxed. If a baby can do it, so can you. Go ahead, try it now. Grab a book (preferably one of mine!) and lie flat on the floor on your back. Put the book on your belly. As you inhale, make the book rise; as you exhale, allow it to drop. Stay there for ten to fifteen minutes to get the hang of it. Once your belly-breathing session is finished, stand up and focus on your breathing. Are you maintaining that belly breathing? I hope so. Try to ALWAYS expand the belly on the inhalation, but do not force it. It should not be forced, but become a natural occurrence. It will become second nature eventually, but it may take awareness and some coaxing. You MUST master this way of breathing for the *Air & Water Diet* to work. Continue with this little exercise for the next few days, months, or years—whatever it takes to change your breathing pattern!

Pay attention to your breathing throughout your day. If it helps your concentration, you can place your hand firmly against your navel while sitting or standing, which will serve the same purpose as the book on the floor. As you inhale, expand your belly to push the hand away. Doing this will serve as a reminder and help you escape from shallow-breathing syndrome.

Another bad habit that inflicts ill effects on the body is holding one's breath. It's just like grunting and stops the oxygen flow. When strong emotions such as anger or fear arise, a person may hold his or her breath without realizing it. You may have caught yourself holding your breath in such a situation, or you may sometimes hold your breath out of habit. I've noticed this in older singers, and it's evident that this change in the breathing pattern can affect metabolism as a person grows older. Don't worry. The habit is probably just a side-effect of sucking in your gut for all those years, and it's easily overcome. Just remember, sucking it in is a sin, and it WILL cause you to hold your breath.

This is a no-brainer. Everyone would rather breathe correctly. Breathing incorrectly—shallow breathing—allows waste to get deposited into our fat cells, which builds more fat cells. But just in case that no-brainer hasn't no-brained you yet, here is a recap of some of the benefits of good breathing.

- Increased energy
- Less stress
- Feeling of calmness
- Improved ability to flush toxins
- Better sleep

- Better skin
- Better self esteem
- Better sex (my favorite)

Now that I got you hot and excited with all this heavy breathing, let's throw some cooling water on the subject.

EATING MORE WATER

I once heard an interviewer ask singer Sebastian Bach about his secret for staying skinny. He said something like, "I just eat water." As funny as that sounds, he was on the right track.

WHY WATER?
Because water is a wonder food, plain and simple. Here's a short list of some of its benefits:

- Regulates body temperature
- Detoxifies the liver
- Helps transport oxygen and nutrients into our cells
- Moisturizes the air in the lung (big plus for singers)
- Increases our metabolism (you should already know this one)
- Moisturizes our joints (thus relieving joint pain)
- Keeps the skin looking younger
- Protects our organs
- Results in clear urine (a sign the kidneys are being taken care of)
- Helps improve the digestive system
- Helps aid bowel function
- Helps flush waste from the system
- Helps shed unwanted pounds (burns fat)
- Enhances the immune system

Are you getting the big picture? By combining the power of air and water, you are opening your body to a whole new world of health. It's sad to think that we've had simple answers to better health and weight control in front of us every day, but we let them slip through our fingers by shallow breathing; holding the breath; and turning to coffee, tea, and soda for our hydration needs. No more, you say? That's music to my ears!

Just for giggles (and to scare the living bejeezus out of you), in case you're still not sold on water, here's a list of what happens when you lack it:

- Lack of energy
- Migraine headaches

- Constipation
- Muscle cramping
- Erratic blood pressure
- Dry skin
- Kidney problems
- Dark yellow urine
- Yellowish phlegm in the throat

If any of the above sounds like you, you may be dehydrated. It's time to rethink your daily water consumption. So, how much water per day, you ask? I'll make it simple.

BODY WEIGHT DIVIDED BY HALF = OUNCES OF WATER PER DAY

It's that easy. If you weigh 200 pounds, you need 100 ounces per day. If you weigh 150, then you need 75. This isn't a morning guzzling extravaganza. You have ALL DAY LONG to drink your quota. Sip, sip, sip is the solution, it's that sippin' simple. Don't worry if you meet your daily water quota three hours before you go to bed. If you're still thirsty, drink more; it won't kill you. (You'd have to consume about ten gallons to perform suicide by aqua.)

Considering that an average of 8 cups of water is lost daily through breathing, perspiration, digestion, and elimination, your daily water quota may not seem like that much compared to what you're losing. So drink up, people!

But don't just drink any water; take pride in the quality of your water. Tap water is a big no-no, at least for me. The water in our neck of the woods (I really do live near the woods) isn't clean enough to water a cat. Okay, I lied, we do water our cats with it; it isn't really all that bad. Let's just say I prefer a slightly cleaner source. You could invest in a water filter for your tap or find a brand of water that you trust is free of BPA (bisphenol A) and other pollutants. BPA, BTW, is a colorless solid that's soluble in organic solvents but poorly soluble in water. It's used to make polycarbonate polymers and epoxy resins, along with other materials used to make plastics, and it has been linked to cancer, infertility, insulin resistance, and miscarriage. It's dangerous stuff. Seek out water that comes in BPA-free containers and also store your water in BPA-free containers. If possible, find a natural spring near your home.

If I don't get water from our local natural spring, I tend to get distilled water. Many will say this is dead water because all its minerals have been removed. I agree. But I'm a clever lad, and I put the minerals right back in, many times over, by adding an X20 packet from singerswater.com. Don't let the "singerswater" fool you. This turns your normal water into singer's water, super water, diet water, and health water, because each sachet of X20 contains calcium, magnesium, and more than 70 trace minerals. These essential minerals and electrolytes become ionic in water, allowing your body to absorb them quickly and easily. I also use the X20 water bottle because it's—wait for it—BPA FREE!

That's enough about water. There is so much information on the Internet about the benefits of water that I suggest you do a little research. If you want to hear me jabber more about water, check out my book *Raise Your Voice*. I wrote enough about water in that book to bore a boar!

That was easy, no? If you change your respiration back to natural breathing (remember those babies!) and adjust your water intake, you'll be on your way to a better day. But hold up a sec, you belly-breathing, water-guzzling wannabe-weight-losing animal. I said it was easy, but it's not *this* easy. It's time to combine air and water for the one-two punch!

LIVING THE AIR & WATER DIET

You should've known you weren't going to get away from me without a little work. Surely you remember "couch potato cardio." I've designed one super-duper simple exercise to keep you drinking more air and eating more water daily. Don't whine, it could've been worse. My *Ultimate Breathing Workout* program contains a nine-exercise system plus a half dozen other specialized breathing exercises to turn you into a breathing machine. Be happy I only stuck you with one!

TABATA BREATHING—THE FOUR-MINUTE FAT-BURNING MIRACLE EXERCISE
Anyone who has read my previous works knows that I love to slip in exercise in all forms, including vocal, breathing, and overall physical conditioning, and my *Mindset* readers already know I'm in love with the notion of "four-minute training." So, to get you up off that couch (or on it, if you prefer; after all, I did dub this "couch potato cardio") and stoking those internal flames, I had to figure out a way—besides simply correcting your bad breathing habits—to get you to do a short burst of cardio to put more oxygen into your system.

I turned to what's called the Tabata Protocol, which was created by Japanese scientist Izumi Tabata while working with his country's Olympic speed skaters. He discovered that athletes using a rotation of short bursts of maximum effort (20 seconds) followed by abbreviated periods of rest (10 seconds), for a period of eight rounds (four minutes total), could achieve better fat-burning, endurance-building results than they could with longer but less-intense workouts.

Imagine getting as intense a workout in four minutes as you'd get in forty-five minutes or an hour. Would that pique your interest? I thought so. But if not, I'll make it even more appealing: I'm not referring to actual exercise; we'll simply conduct four minutes of *Tabata Breathing*, as follows:

1. Extreme panting, 20 seconds
2. Rest while sipping water, 10 seconds
3. Repeat eight times (for a total of four minutes)

WOW, that's easy! All you have to do is pant like a crazy person, and I mean PANT. Superfast, super-expanded inhalation (expand the belly, back, and sides as WIDE as possible), and then a superfast exhalation (deflate that belly, back, and sides as flat as possible) for twenty seconds, then sip water for ten seconds while resting (regular breathing while resting; don't hold your breath), as if it's rising in price like gasoline and you need to take it in like a camel before you go broke! Rinse, lather, repeat.

> **Note:** On that 20th second of panting, you MUST make sure to expel as much breath as you can before beginning your 10-second rest-and-sipping cycle. This quick expulsion action will not only force the abdominals and back muscles to squeeze inward (thus strengthening the muscles) but also help to force stagnant air out of your lungs, thus removing toxins and preparing you for a full, fresh tank of air once you begin panting. This expulsion movement can also cause bad breath because of the stagnant, toxin-filled air you're releasing. You'll taste and smell the difference in the air when you force yourself to release that last bit of stagnant air. Don't worry, just brush your teeth or suck on a mint.

When panting during this exercise, inhale and exhale as deeply and quickly as possible. It should feel like your stomach is a filled water balloon on a full breath and like your belly button is touching your spine on the full exhalation. This tightens and then relaxes the diaphragm, back, and abdominal muscles, toning them in the process. (Guess I lied earlier, we ARE toning a few muscles.) During the 20-second cycle, aim for as many full pants (one pant = one inhalation/exhalation cycle) as possible. You may only get 10 to 20 when starting out, but your ultimate goal should be between 50 and 100 pants. This will wear you out. If it doesn't, you didn't work hard enough. Come on, it's only four minutes.

As for sipping water, you should aim to consume a minimum of 16 ounces during this exercise. It should be easy. More water increases metabolism, fills you up before a meal (so you eat less), and will help flush out more toxins.

Tabata Breathing will help wake you up in the morning, energizing you for a fresh start on your day. In addition, it will help you calm your mind and relax your body right before bedtime (which is great because better sleep = better metabolism). BUT, most importantly, it's a metabolism kick-starter right before your meals. By flooding the body with oxygen and getting more water into your system right before eating, you turn up that fat-burning furnace, aiding digestion and helping to burn off excess calories. It also helps to flush the body of toxins (instead of storing excess fat) through the bowels and kidneys.

Tabata Breathing can be performed on the couch, in bed, on the can, anywhere and everywhere. And BTW, if you own a smart phone, head to your app store to grab the *Tabata Breathing Timer* app (Tabata Breathing Timer) to guide you through this exercise.

Do four minutes seem like too much for all my couch potatoes out there? No problem. You can start with one minute per day and work up four. There's no rush to get to four minutes (but, come on, don't take forever, either). The point is to begin doing it every day. Bottom line, breathing stokes our internal fire. You'll feel flushed from Tabata Breathing, but don't worry. Your flushed skin indicates that you've flooded the body with oxygen and heated up the cells, allowing them to release more garbage and fat. Yay!

WHEN TO PERFORM THIS EXERCISE
Multiple times a day! Perform it when you first wake up and when you need a quick pick-me-up. (Yes, it will give you a boost of energy.) Perform it before going to bed, and above all, ALWAYS perform this exercise right before eating every snack and every meal. The increased oxygen and water intake will aid digestion, thus nipping the fat-building culprit in the bud before it spreads like weeds. So, one more time, perform this simple breathing/drinking exercise:

- Upon waking
- Before eating (and after your meal helps too)
- When you need a boost of energy
- Before bedtime

When you wake up, grab your Tabata Breathing Timer and a glass of water, and breathe, sip, breathe. Repeat right before breakfast, lunch, and dinner. And for a big fat-burning bonus, repeat the exercise right after your meal to aid digestion even more. Don't forget to finish your day with this exercise just as you're retiring to bed. Yes, you may pee once or twice during the night, but it helps flush your kidneys and keeps the lungs moist.

> **Note:** For those of you who also perform the mind/body process from my book *Unleash Your Creative Mindset*, simply perform the Tabata Breathing exercise first.

Now you're on your own. Correct your breathing, adjust your water quota to match your current weight, and start performing the Tabata Breathing exercise throughout the day when required. I guarantee you'll begin to feel better, leaner, and meaner within a month! But I don't want to leave you high and dry, so I've added just a few more pages to keep you moving forward with your new way of life. Read on.

PROGRAM REVIEW

The following isn't required, but it sure would help. Since we're so addicted to junk food, I thought I'd share a way to help reset the body by getting more air and water into us through our food. The best way to accomplish this is a seven-day juice fast, consuming juice (instead of solid food) for every meal. It consists of the following:

Meal (Breakfast/Lunch/Dinner)
- Four to six leaves of kale
- Handful of spinach
- Half-inch to 1 inch of ginger
- Four stalks of celery
- Two apples (red or green)
- Half lemon, squeezed

Snack (as needed)
- Three apples
- Two large carrots
- Handful of blueberries

Note: To ensure that you're getting the highest-quality food that's free of pesticides, ALWAYS purchase organic fruits and vegetables when available.

A juice fast will give the digestive system a break and get you away from junk food and all that processed food full of white salt, sugar, and flour. Continue meeting your daily water quota as well as performing your regular Tabata Breathing sessions.

This fast is great for singers. If you're a singer and you decide to follow this juice regimen for a week, please add pineapple juice, as bromelain is beneficial for the voice. And add an ounce of aloe vera juice, too. Remember, go organic whenever possible.

You may experience tiredness and headaches during the fast, but stay strong. If you feel hungry, drink more juice.

FYI—In the past, I've used a Jack LaLanne juicer, but it's extremely messy. I've since switched to a Breville compact juicer. It's only slightly messy (there's no getting around a bit of mess when you juice, but it's worth it), and there are fewer components to clean. It cost less than one hundred dollars.

Once you've completed the seven-day juice-fast reset, you should consider sticking with juice to replace at least one meal per day. You'll notice that certain cravings (such as caffeine and sugar cravings) begin to diminish. Stay away from what caused that craving in the first place. Replace your sweet cravings with fruits. Replace coffee and cola with water. Add veggies to your plate and eat less processed bread! Your body will thank you!

Juicing and fruit and veggie snacking resets your metabolism. Think of fruits and veggies as high quality "air and water food" and everything else (processed foods, white sugar, flour, water, red meats) as, well, less efficient in the air and water department. We are incredibly adaptive creatures, and our bodies adapt to how and what we eat. Eat junk, and you'll look and feel like junk. Eat healthy and juice, and you'll regain the energy of your youth! I've tried various diets before, even some that can put strain on the heart. I once lost 11 pounds in 4 days, but as soon as I went off that crazy diet, I gained the weight back in a matter of days. The *Air & Water Diet,* juicing, and adding more fruits and veggies to your daily food consumption is not a diet, but a way of life, a better, healthier way of life. Change your lifestyle and live more healthfully.

Don't forget to supplement. I won't turn this into to a vitamin/herb/mineral book, as I've written other books that cover that subject. But do some research to make sure you're also getting your vitamins and minerals (though juicing will help).

And finally, duh, duh, duh, EXERCISE. Don't let that word scare you. Sure, Tabata Breathing is awesome, but what if we upped our workout a notch? The best way for Tabata Breathers to up the ante is to add four minutes of skipping rope using the Tabata protocol. A four-minute rope-skipping session every day will knock your socks off, trust me! All you need to do is a basic jump-rope pattern, with the feet close together. If you're a pro jumper, you can change it up, alternating leg lifts, as if you're running as you skip rope. There are many ways to skip rope, so challenge yourself. If you have joint problems and the force of landing on the ground taxes the hips, knees, or ankles, I have a solution. Skip rope while bouncing on a rebounder—you know, one of those mini trampolines. This will make each landing much softer, but skipping on a rebounder WILL slow it down. But as long as you're working hard, it will be just as effective.

If you decide to add Tabata Skipping to your routine, do as follows:

- One round of Tabata Breathing
- One round of Tabata Protocol (jump rope weapon of choice)

If you don't have a real jump rope, buy one. I like the cheap licorice jump ropes because they're so compact I can throw them in my laptop briefcase and always have it with me when I'm on the road. A speed rope, segmented rope, or weighted rope is also fine. If you want to start this program today, but you don't have your jump rope yet, pretend you have one. Don't let "I don't have a jump rope" be an excuse. Grab two handfuls of air and swing your arms like a crazy person. Speaking of crazy, you REALLY want to wear yourself out during this exercise. If you thought you were tired after Tabata Breathing, you've got a big surprise coming. Attempt a minimum of 50 skips during each twenty-second cycle, building toward 100 skips per cycle. Your heart will race and threaten to leap out of your chest, like the newborn monster in *Alien*. (In space, no one can hear you pant.) Don't worry, your ribs will keep it in. So skip like crazy, don't be lazy! If you're not tired at the end of four minutes, well, as I said for Tabata Breathing, *You didn't work hard enough.*

Though I strongly recommend that you skip for this workout, your exercise choices are limitless. If skipping doesn't do it for you, try something else. Jumping jacks, burpees, sit-ups, and squats work well, or combine them all from my "Maximizer" exercise as explained in my book *Raise Your Voice 2: The Advanced Manual*. Be forewarned: It's a beast and only for those of you ready to surpass couch potato cardio.

There you have it, simple enough to keep you doing the program without scratching your head. The *Air & Water Diet* in a nutshell is:

Required
- Breathe correctly.
- Meet your daily water quota.
- Perform Tabata Breathing as required.

Bonus
- Eat more fruits and veggies (because they're naturally full of air and water).
- If you're tough enough, try a seven-day juice fast.
- If you're even tougher, add more exercise (Tabata skipping, Maximizer, etc.). If you're the toughest, double your workout to sixteen minutes. One round of Tabata Breathing, one round of Tabata Skipping, and two rounds of two different exercises (burpees, pushups, situps, etc.).

It's time to get busy. I can't make this book any shorter or this program any simpler. See you on the skinny scales. But, before you hit those scales, I'd like to add that if you feel you're becoming an extreme-breathing, water-drinking addict, you may also enjoy my books *Raise Your Voice Second Edition*, *Raise Your Voice 2: The Advanced Manual*, and *The Ultimate Breathing Workout*. All three books go into deeper detail concerning breathing, water intake, diet, and exercise. Good luck on your new life adventure!

Jaime Vendera

PractiSING

Do you know that the No. 1 secret to vocal success and the No. 1 roadblock in a singer's path to vocal success are one and the same? And it's not what you might think. It isn't talent, skill, intonation, charisma, or any other attribute you might possess or lack. It is simply "practice." Practice is the two-sided coin that leads to success or failure. With practice, you can rise to greatness, but without it, you'll never reach the next rung on the ladder. I know that practice is the key, because I've seen the results of practice lift singers to great heights, and I've watched other singers plummet to the bottom by avoiding it.

Practice leads to perfection, plain and simple. With my experience training thousands of singers since 1996, I know this to be true. My most successful students live and breathe their vocal exercises and love to rehearse their song repertoire, while my least successful students ... well, I'm skeptical when they tell me they practice at all. I know when a singer has practiced; their progress reveals the truth, and it's easy to deduce when a lazy singer has put in a sparse ten minutes a day once or twice per week, if that much.

You can read a book on singing, watch a zillion videos, study your favorite singer, attend a vocal workshop, or take a vocal lesson, but unless you put what you've learned into practical application through repetition, you'll never reap the benefits.

"But I've done all this stuff, Jaime, and I am STILL not getting any better at singing!"

Believe it or not, there ARE singers who consume all things vocal-related. They learn the latest terminology, usually ridiculous, but often smart sounding. They study every vocal methodology on the planet with great intensity, claiming to have mastered their vocal technique through magical mental osmosis. They have become one with the voice, able to write a dissertation on why a certain vocal exercise does what it does, how the diaphragm works, and how the narrowing of the glottis and thinning of the vocal cords enables one to sing high notes in full voice. But all that information is only stored in their heads, not fully explored through their own voice. The voice and the body must experience what the mind has ingested, and only through repetition of an activity will you become better at it.

I've wracked my brains for years wondering why some students cringe at the thought of putting in the practice time to become better singers. I've pondered how to inspire my students to work beyond this procrastination-driven vocal block, to develop the same burning desire that I had when I started. But, after writing and creating dozens of books, videos, and audio programs; performing on countless television shows; conducting vocal workshops around the world; and even creating an online vocal school, I still hadn't found the answer. Yet my mind was and is always at work, constantly seeking new ways to perfect this art form we call singing.

My persistence paid off. I fell asleep one night pondering how to enlighten a group of my students from the Vendera Vocal Academy through new, intense ways of practicing my vocal exercises. The Academy was growing, and I would soon be creating the second-year curriculum. I knew I had to take their voice-strengthening regimen to a new level. This is my usual process whenever I need to unleash new creative thoughts. I program my mind to tap into my creative mindset via the techniques from my book *Unleash Your Creative Mindset*, which helps me subconsciously attack a problem in need of a solution throughout the day and while I sleep. I fell asleep with thoughts of my students, and as I slept, vivid dreams about practice raced through my head. Some old ideas and some new ones visited my dreams that night, and I awoke with a new fire! As I jotted down the new ideas in my Mindset Journal (so I wouldn't forget what I had dreamed), it dawned on me that I had actually discovered the solution to other singers' problems, a way to tear down the wall of procrastination preventing them from practicing.

The answer seemed so simple that I was shocked I hadn't thought of it sooner. I was angry with myself for not addressing the issue years before. I'd known for a decade that practice was problematic for many singers. I'd known from personal experience that the percentage of students who rarely practiced my methods after learning the techniques and exercises was far greater than the percentage of students who did practice. I'd known it didn't matter whether a student had read my books, attended my online school, the Vendera Vocal Academy, or studied with me personally; the outcome was the same—practice, for most, usually fell short.

PROCRASTINATION ELIMINATION

Before we can change the way we practice, we must first get to the root cause of WHY we're not practicing the way we should. You might be saying, "Jaime, I DO practice some, I practice when I can find the time, blah, blah, blah ..." Any excuse you throw at me for not practicing, I've already heard. Excuses are weak ways of mentally justifying the avoidance of practice and placing the blame onto anyone or anything besides yourself. So, you missed your practice session because your day was so busy with regular life that you couldn't find time to spend on your voice. This is faulty reasoning. The "I can't practice because" list of excuses is simply another form of vocal abuse. I'm not trying to point fingers or upset you, I'm just being honest. Excuses are vocal abuse because you're hurting your voice by not allowing it to grow stronger.

The best way to overcome these excuses is to acknowledge that we've created them and then face them head on. We need to figure out the core reason behind each excuse so that we can overcome the power it holds over us. Following is a list of fifteen excuses, fifteen reasons we procrastinate when it comes to vocal exercise. There are many more excuses, but this list covers the general excuses I've heard from singers over the years. If ANY of the following reasons ring true in your own life, whether one, seven, or all fifteen, please write each excuse down on a sheet of paper to recall exactly which ones are hampering your ability to practice. Once you've honestly accepted which of the fifteen excuses relate to you, we can address each excuse and overcome its power over us:

- I don't know how to practice.
- Practicing is boring.
- I'm too tired to practice.
- I just don't feel like practicing right now.
- I don't need to practice as much as other singers.
- I can always practice more tomorrow.
- I'd rather be singing.
- I've got plenty of time today to finish my exercises.
- I'll just have to do it again tomorrow.
- I can't come up with a good enough reason to practice.
- Practice can wait.
- If I wait until tonight, I'll practice right before I go to bed.
- I just can't find the time for practice.

- I never get any better when I practice.
- When I do the exercises, they hurt my singing voice, so why do them?

How many of the above excuses did you write down on your list? Or were you 100% free and clear from excuse abuse? Come on, be honest with yourself. If you truly want to overcome procrastination and practice more efficiently, it starts with being honest with yourself and addressing the excuses that affect you. Read the list one more time and admit to yourself whether any of the excuses ring true. It doesn't matter how many strike a chord, we CAN overcome each excuse. I'm about to show you exactly HOW to destroy all your excuses by reviewing each excuse and destroying the rationalization and power you give to each of them.

I DON'T KNOW HOW OR WHAT TO PRACTICE

One of the top excuses I hear for not practicing is, "I'm just not sure how or what to practice." Many singers claim to be confused about the "how" or "what" of practicing. If you're confused, it's simple to fix. ASK YOUR VOCAL COACH! If that coach is me, you've got plenty of books, videos, audio programs, Skype lessons, and an actual online vocal school to back you up, so there is NO excuse for using this excuse!

Do you want to know exactly what exercises to perform each day and how to perform them correctly? Just ask! At the Vendera Vocal Academy, I lay out a practice regimen week by week. There is no second-guessing; you know EXACTLY what you must practice. Moreover, in each of my books I lay out a precise regimen. For example, in books like *Raise Your Voice*, *Sing Out Loud*, *SingFit*, and *Ultimate Breathing Workout*, I always present precise instructions on what exercises must be performed and how to perform them correctly. In each book, I explain why they work and how to approach vocal technique as you perform the exercise. I encourage each singer to use a diary to keep track of progress, and I ask them to check off each exercise as they perform it daily.

There is no excuse for not knowing what to practice or how to practice. If you don't know what or how, ask your vocal coach. Hopefully, it's me, ha-ha. If you don't have a vocal coach, buy a book, watch an instructional video, or listen to audio programs to learn the basics. Then you can create your own daily vocal training program. You won't know what or how until you ask your coach and study. Drop the excuse and start researching this subject to develop your vocal routine.

PRACTICING IS BORING

Practice is only boring because you're making it boring. If you truly lack the desire and don't have a clear vision of your future vocal goals, then yes, it might be boring. YOU have to find that excitement to drive away the boredom you are experiencing. I don't know about you, but whenever I would practice and discover new notes in my range or new vocal tones and realize that my voice was growing, I was ten kinds of excited. Maybe you experienced that same excitement when you hit a high note for the first time. But perhaps you couldn't find your way back to that high note, so the excitement faded away. That's when you let the boredom creep in. This is typical, because we generally seek continual confirmation that we're improving. That sudden high from reaching a new note not only provides confirmation but also creates a feeling of elation that we yearn to experience with every note that leaves our mouths. If we don't constantly experience that elation, we sometimes develop the "I want it now" syndrome, and since we don't experience that singer's high during every minute of practice, we have a tendency to lose interest. The key is to remember that elated moment, to close our eyes and experience how it made us feel, to cherish it and hold on to it, to imagine it DOES happen every moment, and be like an excited child the night before Christmas, expecting it to happen again. Yearn for it, strive for it, and it will return. Hanging on to that moment will help you find the excitement of practice.

I'M TOO TIRED TO PRACTICE

Poor baby. Let me tell you about true exhaustion. I used to work construction. One summer, during a monster heat wave, I experienced extreme health issues. The sun had affected my skin and my heart, and I would leave work super exhausted, feeling like I was about to die and my heart was about to pop out of my chest. And then I would rehearse with a band two hours a night, three times per week. If I can do it, so can you. If you're always striving to reach that elated feeling, practice will actually give you a second wind. Many coaches recommend not practicing when you're tired, but I say it's the perfect time to focus on your technique so you support your voice when the rest of your body lacks energy. Riddle me this: What are you going to do when you're on the road supporting your No.1 hit and you're just "too tired" to perform for 50,000 screaming fans? Are you going to whine about it and tell the promoters that you need some sleepy time? I didn't think so. Tired or not, ALWAYS practice like you've already made it big and your next concert is tonight.

I JUST DON'T FEEL LIKE PRACTICING RIGHT NOW

I guess you don't feel like having a great voice either! If you use this excuse, you don't want it bad enough and should probably quit right now. Just forget all about all this singing crap. Don't like my answer? Then shut up, quit complaining, and start feeling like it this instant to prove that you DO want to be an amazing singer! Winners train, losers complain! Are you a winner or a loser?

I DON'T NEED TO PRACTICE AS MUCH AS OTHER SINGERS
Do you honestly think you're better than other singers? You might be better than some—maybe—but there is always someone better ready to take your place. Are you ready to give up your place in line? If your attitude is "I'm already a great singer, I have more range than so and so," and you think that's a good excuse not to practice as much as other singers, you're dead wrong. You've let your ego take control. IF, by some chance, you are a bit better than your average singer, congratulations; it means you must practice even harder than the others to maintain your current singing level. When people hear you they will expect you to sound great, and the only way to maintain great range and power is to practice even more. Consider a bodybuilder who has built a massive chest. It takes that bodybuilder more weight to keep all that muscle. If you practice less, you will lose that muscle! The better you become, the more practice it takes to keep you there.

I CAN ALWAYS PRACTICE MORE TOMORROW
Yep, you sure can, but now you've lost a day where you might have made an amazing vocal breakthrough. You've thrown away a practice session that could have catapulted you to the next level. At the end of this book, when we cover the Percentage Deduction Technique, you'll see just how important NOT waiting until tomorrow can be towards vocal progress.

I'D RATHER BE SINGING
Yes, this is true; we all would rather be singing. But singing is not the same as performing vocal exercises for voice strengthening. Though singing helps make you a better singer by improving your art, vocal strength training allows you to gain control over your technique as you build muscle so that when you do sing, your voice flows naturally without strain, allowing your artistic interpretation of each song to bloom.

I'VE GOT PLENTY OF TIME TODAY TO FINISH MY EXERCISES
I hear this one a lot. You promise yourself you'll practice first thing in the morning, but you get too busy checking your email. You talk yourself into practicing in the afternoon, which is interrupted by a soap opera and a call from your long-lost high school buddy. Practice time is shoved off until the wee hours of the evening, which you forget about until your head hits the pillow. So you re-use the "I'll practice tomorrow" excuse, and then, BAM, it's the next day, which means you missed yet another day of practice. This excuse won't even exist by the end of this book, because *PractiSing* requires that you vocalize early, and I mean early, in the morning. So go ahead, hang on to this one until the end of the chapter, because it's not gonna stick for long.

IF I WAIT UNTIL TONIGHT, I'LL PRACTICE RIGHT BEFORE I GO TO BED

This excuse is really a hybrid child of the last excuse, but it has a different reasoning behind it. Many singers believe their voices are at their best later in the day. That's a myth that I'm going to disprove. Many singers hate to sing first thing in the morning, claiming their voices aren't awake. Yes, your voice does need to wake up, but a great warm-up will have you ready to sing first thing in the morning. I've sung songs by Led Zeppelin, Nazareth, Alice in Chains, and my own songs on television shows in the wee hours of the morning without fear of my voice not being "awake." With practice, great singers can sing whenever, and that's how we'll attack the practice philosophy in this book. So, no more late-night practice sessions, unless it's an extra session on top of what you did earlier in the day. Personally, I don't believe in the late-night practice session as our only session, because our minds are so filled with the emotions and memories of the day that we tend to not focus on the exercises. We also risk skipping our routine altogether, becoming too involved in a television show, coming home late after a dinner out, or searching the Internet. We may wind up too sleepy to follow through with our vocal exercises. If you're a late-night-practice type, it's time to change up your routine.

I'LL JUST HAVE TO DO IT AGAIN TOMORROW

And the next day, and the next day, and the next ... Listen, if you HATE practicing, then this excuse is the easy cop-out. Winners train, losers complain. I found a T-shirt with this motto, so I had to buy it and wear it in several of my Vendera Vocal Academy training videos. I want ALL of my singers to be winners who train. Think of your vocal practice routine as a way of life, as much a part of you as eating, drinking, breathing, and sleeping. You ARE your instrument, therefore you MUST train your instrument daily. Enough said!

I CAN'T COME UP WITH A GOOD ENOUGH REASON TO PRACTICE

You're telling me that practice just doesn't work for you, doesn't fit your lifestyle. *Ding-ding-ding*, congratulations, you are the ultimate procrastinator, so you deserve the Biggest Loser Award, and I'm not talkin' 'bout the TV show. If you're weighing the pros and the cons, and you've used all these other excuses to tip the scales in your lazy favor, then you've just talked yourself out of greatness. You only need one good excuse to practice, and I've got it, and hey, it's a great excuse! The only reason you need for practicing is to become an amazing singer! Nuff said! Again, how bad do you want it? *Proooove* it!

PRACTICE CAN WAIT
Practice CANNOT wait. Your time is now! It is of the utmost urgency that you practice here, there, everywhere—but only if you want to be amazing. Put in the time and I guarantee you'll be amazing, and then you'll finally understand that practice can never wait, practice happens in every minute of the day. Any time you take a breath and exhale, you could have turned that exhalation into a vocal exercise. One more time: How bad do you want it?

I JUST CAN'T FIND THE TIME FOR PRACTICE
It's the procrastinator's lullaby. I hear this one more than I hear my own name. "But, Jaime, my job keeps me too busy, I have school work, I'm dealing with the kids, I got to help my buddy move into his apartment, I have football practice, the cheerleading squad meets after school, I have to study for the next Mathlete tournament ..." The list goes on and on. You'll never be able to find time to practice if that's your mindset. Winners MAKE time to practice. You can find time slots to practice all throughout your day, before you leave the house in the morning, while driving to work, during a lunch break, while cooking dinner, right after school on your walk or ride home, etc. Though you'll soon see that the best practice time is first thing in the morning, my goal is to turn you into a walking vocal exercise so that you utilize every possible moment to become a better, stronger singer.

I NEVER GET ANY BETTER WHEN I PRACTICE
This could almost be a legitimate excuse, because vocal improvement does take time, and it may seem as if you aren't getting any better through certain periods of your vocal journey. Don't sweat it if your vocal growth seems to have halted for a week or two. Don't get discouraged. You'll grow soon enough if you stick with your routine. However, if you've been faithfully practicing for months and months and you're still stuck in the same vocal spot, there may be reasons for it. The problem might be your approach to vocal technique, the way you're performing your exercises, or even the guidance of your current vocal coach. I've had coaches that hampered my abilities and stifled my growth. In fact, this very morning a new student from China told me he's had forty to fifty vocal lessons, most recently sixteen lessons with the same coach, yet he cannot sing any higher than the A above middle C. I had him singing the B above middle C within 40 minutes. So, yes, sometimes this excuse is a legitimate one. But you have to decide WHY this excuse applies to you. Are you just plateauing for a spell or is it something deeper, such as a misunderstanding of vocal technique or misguidance from a vocal coach. Or is it lack of practice? If you started practicing two weeks ago and you're only practicing your routine three to four days a week and you still aren't improving, the problem is simple—

you lack something called patience. Get back to work and be patient! Perfection takes time!

WHEN I DO THE EXERCISES, THEY HURT MY SINGING VOICE, SO WHY DO THEM?
Again, this excuse could be legitimate and for many of the same reasons. Your voice could hurt if you're confused about vocal technique and don't know how to correctly perform each exercise. It could be the result of poor guidance from a vocal coach. It could be that you're going at it like a wild animal, with no remorse for your poor little vocal cords, slamming the bejeezus out of them in order to hit the same notes as your favorite singer when you're not quite there yet. YOU have to decide what is causing the pain. Bottom line, if it hurts, stop, because you're doing something wrong. Re-evaluate your approach to vocal technique and your approach to your practice sessions.

I've summed up my thoughts and feelings on each excuse. Now we must discover how to erase these excuses from our minds in order to focus on better vocal practice etiquette. How do we do that? It's a simple yet effective technique that begins with the mind, which I have dubbed the Mirror Mindset technique. First, you turn each negative excuse into a positive statement. Then, every morning at 5 a.m. (YES, I said 5 a.m.!) you get your singing butt up out of bed, stand in front of a mirror, look directly into your eyes as if talking to yourself, and recite each positive statement three times in a row. If you had three excuses, you now have three new positive statements that you must recite to yourself in front of a mirror three times each. This technique is based on the experience I had on my very first television show, *Good Morning America*, when I was having trouble breaking glass. If you've read my other books, you'll recall that I spent many times in front of a mirror, which I am sure (with help from GOD, of course) changed the path of my life by making that first performance very successful. So, if you're ready to erase all of those excuses from your mind and vocabulary, here are your new positive statements:

I don't know how to practice =
I now know exactly how and what to practice

Practicing is boring =
Practice is exciting

I'm too tired to practice =
Practicing gives me my second wind

I just don't feel like practicing right now =
I'm so anxious to practice

I don't need to practice as much as other singers =
I must practice more than others to reach and maintain my vocal potential

I can always practice more tomorrow =
My time to practice is now

I'd rather be singing =
I love vocalizing before singing

I've got plenty of time today to finish my exercises =
The time for practice is always first thing in the morning

I'll just have to do it again tomorrow =
I cannot wait to practice again tomorrow

I can't come up with a good enough reason to practice =
The reason I practice is to become a better singer

Practice can wait =
Practice can never wait because it's part of my life

If I wait until tonight, I'll practice right before I go to bed =
Morning is the best time for practice

I don't have enough time for practice =
I always make time to practice

I never get any better when I practice =
I get better with each practice session and I know that perfection takes time

When I do the exercises, they hurt my singing voice, so why do them? =
My vocal exercises make my voice feel great

So, you see, I've pulled the veil from all your excuses and given you a way to erase them all, which means NO MORE EXCUSES. Remember, to break the hold these excuses have over your mind, perform the Mirror Mindset technique. Simply change each excuse into its positive counterpart (and write them down to remember them). Look directly into your own eyes while standing in front of a mirror at 5 a.m. each morning, and repeat each counterpart three times in a row, as if you're having a conversation with yourself.

This process will change your mindset. Speaking of which, it would also help if you were performing the Mind/Body process from my book *Unleash Your Creative Mindset*, which will further program your mind for success. But that is optional. Now that we're starting to erase all these excuses, let's move on to a vocal self-evaluation to discover your current vocal abilities and decide where you wish to take your voice.

VOCAL SELF-EVALUATION

You're conquering and erasing your excuses, and you may even be eager to tackle practice again. But first you need to evaluate your own voice. Where are you at vocally right now and where do you want to go with your voice? In other words, how good a singer are you today, and how good a singer do you want to be in the future? Vocal evaluation is one of the main reasons that I created VenderaVocalAcademy.com. I offer a sort of vocal self-evaluation through vocal critiques, which is part of Academy tuition for all singers. The purpose of the critiques is not only to help singers but also to get singers thinking about the outcome of the critique in order to instill self-evaluation. Self-evaluation will let you know where you stand today and give you an idea of where you can go with your voice in the future. Our goal is to figure all of this out and then create a sort of map to guide you toward your destination.

HOW'S MY VOICE NOW?
We're going to conduct two tests to see where your voice is now. The first test is the range test. If you have an iPhone or iPad, my app TUNED XD will become your new best friend, because it is THE digital vocal coach that you can carry with you everywhere. All you need to do to perform this test is a simple vocal slide down in your range on a "Yah" as in "Father" while watching the tuner on TUNED XD. Slide all the way down in your range to find your lowest note. Vocal fry does not count. You're looking for your absolute lowest comfortable note that is audible and solid without any of that vocal fry grit sound; you know, that groggy morning voice. Check the tune to make note of the actual pitch and octave.

Once you've found your lowest note, repeat the "Yah" slide going up in range to find your highest full voice note (not your falsetto). If your voice cracks, you must figure out the exact note where the crack (vocal break) occurred. This is your highest full voice note without forcing your voice higher, which will cause vocal strain.

Your lowest note to your highest is your current usable range in full voice, so you now have an idea of how many notes you can safely and easily use in your singing voice. You may notice that you cannot sing this low or high in a song. While sliding on an open vowel does give you an idea of your vocal range potential from your lowest to your highest note at this moment in time, singing regularly to stretch the voice to those extreme low and high notes is the key to unlocking that full potential. And yes, I know you can go lower on vocal fry, belt out a few higher notes in full voice, possibly go another octave in falsetto, but we're not concerned with those elements in this test. Those who have read my books know that I am a range freak and believe you can go much lower and higher. Not to fret, that will all come in time.

The second test is the song self-critique. I want you to grab Karaoke tracks of two songs you currently sing on a regular basis. These are two very specific songs: the one you consider the easiest for you to sing and the one you consider most challenging. Record yourself singing along to each Karaoke track. TUNED XD users can import the Karaoke tracks and sing along via the two-track practice recorder, which allows you to save your recordings. I expect both songs to be in one take. If you flub the words, sure, I'll let you take a second crack at it, but, bottom line, we want the raw you. Once both songs are recorded, listen back to each song. Critique your performance and make a list of the likes and dislikes of your rendition of each song. Save these recordings and label them by song name and date, because once you have been *PractiSing* for one month, I want you to conduct another song self-critique for each one. You'll compare those to your first song self-critique, and I guarantee you'll notice a huge difference. Song self-critiquing is a great way to improve your singing skills.

WHAT ARE MY VOCAL GOALS?

Now that you've critiqued your voice and made a list of your likes and dislikes, it is time to discuss your vocal goals. I hope that by listening back to each song, you've formulated some new vocal goals. If you strained to belt out the high note in one of your songs, maybe you wish you had more range. Or maybe you want to improve your vibrato. It's time to put your goals down on paper, to turn them into tangible entities. What do want to accomplish with your voice? More range, more stamina, learning to add grit? Your answer will help to line out your actual vocal routine, to help you decide which exercises are best suited to your voice to help reach your vocal goals. We can then transfer these goals into a vocal road map.

CREATING A VOCAL SUCCESS ROAD MAP

Now that you have an idea of your vocal goals, you need a program that will get you there. All my fans and friends know I am probably the most humble vocal coach you'll ever meet, but I'm going to make a suggestion here. My book *Raise Your Voice* and the Vendera Vocal Academy have great vocal success rates. I'm very adamant when it comes to lining out simple, effective vocal training routines that are presented in a way that simplifies vocal technique regardless of whether you want to sing pop, country, blues, gospel, rock, metal and whether you want to sing lower, higher, cleaner, grittier, softer, louder, or breathier. We have exercises for all of it. I suggest you start with *Raise Your Voice* or join the Vendera Vocal Academy.

FYI: If you join the Academy, you receive a free copy of the *Raise Your Voice* eBook as well as a free 15-minute vocal warm-up MP3 routine and a free downloadable practice journal to help keep track of your progress. So, the road map will be lined out for you. If you want to add things like grit exercises, breathing exercises, vibrato exercises, etc., based on your goals, they are covered in *Raise Your Voice* and at the Vendera Vocal Academy as well.

Just so you aren't confused, your vocal road map is simply your daily plan, written down on paper. It first lists your goals, followed by a list of your vocal exercises, cardio routines, diet regimen, etc. It's written down so you can review it daily to remind yourself what exercises need to be performed to reach your vocal goal. It can simply be a few notes on your iPhone, such as:

"Since I want more range and stamina for stage, every day I must perform Jaime Vendera's Ultimate Vocal Warm Up to prepare my voice and then perform his three Isolation exercises, followed by a run on a treadmill while singing for 45 minutes."

There, I have created a super-simple basic map of my daily routine, which reminds me that I want more range and vocal stamina, and to gain this range and stamina, I must warm up and then practice three vocal exercises before running on a treadmill while singing some songs.

You've overcome your excuses, self-evaluated your voice, and decided on your vocal goals. You've created your vocal road map, thus choosing which exercises to perform daily. Congratulations. Now it's time to dive into the true *PractiSing* ideology.

PRACTISING APPLICATION

In case you haven't quite figured it out yet, I've already started you on the *PractiSing* program. You see, the first step to the art of *PractiSing* is starting your day at the early hour of 5 a.m. Since you've already been up performing your Mirror Mindset technique at 5 a.m., you're somewhat prepared for that early morning rise. So let's discuss why 5 a.m. is so important.

VOCALIZING AT 5 A.M.

For some reason, starting at 5 a.m., before the sun rises, seems to be the best time to get in your vocal workout routine as well as your cardio and weight lifting. Your mind is alert but just waking up, and not cluttered with the worries of the day. Thus, you're better able to focus on your vocal exercises. You'll discover that practice in the early morning flies by quicker than at any other time of day. So, first thing you do in the morning is the mirror technique, and then off to practice in your car, your basement, the shower, a garage, wherever you need to practice to be alone and not disturb the rest of the family. When I wrote *Raise Your Voice*, I was practicing before 5 a.m. while driving to work. Starting my day with my vocal and physical routine allows me to accomplish much more. In addition, I feel much more satisfied once I'm finished with my vocal and physical exercises, because I don't have to worry throughout the rest of the day about how/when/where I'll "find the time" to get in my vocal exercises, ha-ha.

I've seen books written about the magical hour of 5 a.m. and know for myself it's true. Be aware that for the first week or two, your voice may seem to hate you for starting your vocal workout so early in the morning. Stick with it; your voice will come around, and then you'll be amazed at the difference it makes, not only in building a better voice but also in your attitude toward vocal practice. Once you're in the flow, your vocal exercises will almost be on auto-pilot and you'll start loving, not despising, practice. By knocking those exercises out when you first wake up, you're beating that procrastinator in the back of your mind to the punch. By the time you're finished vocalizing, that procrastinator has nothing left to procrastinate about.

KEEPING A VOCAL WORKOUT JOURNAL

Now that you're up at 5 a.m. doing your thing, I also want you to keep a vocal journal. You already wrote down your excuses and turned them into something positive, and you also wrote down a vocal road map, so why not keep a workout journal, too? Those of you who have read any of my books, such as *Raise Your Voice*, *Raise Your Voice 2: The Advanced Manual*, *SingFit*, or *Unleash Your Creative Mindset* know that I am a diary/journal freak. I created a book called *The Ultimate Vocal Workout Diary* and talk about the Mindset Diary in *Unleash Your Creative Mindset*. I have a specific vocal workout journal in *SingFit* because I truly believe that one of the best ways to overcome procrastination and ignite the desire fire within is to make yourself responsible for completing your daily vocal routine and other tasks by keeping track of each exercise, your diet, song repertoire, etc., in a vocal workout journal. So, now that you've decided which exercises to perform (hopefully mine, ha-ha), review your vocal road map and list each exercise on a sheet of paper in what will become your vocal workout journal. (If you wish, you can use *The Ultimate Vocal Workout Diary*.) You can either check off the exercise daily upon completion or elaborate further by listing your lowest/highest note for each exercise so you can also track your range increase.

THE 10,000 CHALLENGE

There is more to overcoming the practice blues than waking up at 5 a.m. and checking off each exercise as you complete it. Getting up at 5 a.m. IS a major part of beating procrastination, but wait, there's more—the REAL trick to making *PractiSing* a way of life is performing the 10,000 Challenge. The best part of the dream that evolved into this book was discovering the 10,000 Challenge. I woke up thinking about my Academy students, and I was pondering ways to make them strive for more, when a little voice whispered, "They need to repeat each exercise 10,000 times." Then I remembered my dream, seeing myself performing each of my exercises: 10,000 Lip Bubbles, 10,000 Resonant Hums, 10,000 Gargling Tones, 10,000 Falsetto Slides, 10,000 Transcending Tones, and 10,000 Sirens. Then I recalled a saying I had heard many times before, that it takes 10,000 hours to master anything, a slam dunk, a home run, etc. Days after my dream, synchronicity caused my coach, Jim Gillette, to mention that I should read the book *Outliers: The Story of Success* by Malcolm Gladwell. Malcolm searched for a master and discovered something very interesting. It took 10,000 hours of practice to master anything. None of the masters he found had less than 10,000 hours dedicated to their chosen profession. So, 10,000 seemed like a magical number.

My creative mindset formulated a unique way to use this magical number to "master" an individual vocal exercise in far less than 10,000 hours. I drove myself stinking mad wanting to repeat each exercise 10,000 times. Again, this was part of my dream and something I have since developed for Year Two Vendera Vocal Academy students. Each training session in Year Two presents a new 10,000 Challenge for a specific exercise on top of their regular exercise routine. These 10,000 rep challenges are conducted with very simple exercises, such as a Lip Bubble Slide, a Siren, or a Falsetto Slide, without worrying about the pitch, just randomly performing reps of them throughout the day. I used this same approach (though I didn't count my reps) years ago when I worked construction. While building a heart and vascular building for a hospital, I would perform a hybrid Falsetto Slide Siren wail, and I had my entire crew screaming along. The more we all wailed, the stronger, louder, and higher our unified voices became. It got so intense that someone at the hospital wrote a letter to my office stating, "It has come to our attention that foreman Jaime Vendera is creating loud siren noises. They are so loud that they are scaring some of our outpatients and confusing our staff as to when an actual ambulance is arriving. Could you please ask Mr. Vendera to refrain from making these noises?"

I was little cocky back then, so I continued wailing, determined to get even louder and higher, ha-ha. How did they retaliate? They knew I had appeared on *MythBusters* the year before, so they asked me if I would break a wineglass at the dinner in honor of the new building. If you go to YouTube.com/venderaj and search for "Tarzan Vendera," you can watch the actual clip from the performance. (FYI—I'm not making the Tarzan scream. I was so loud that I knocked out their microphone feed, so they stuck a little Tarzan scream in just for fun.)

Long story short, my high, piercing notes were eerie powerful. Coming full circle years later, I remembered the power of performing one simple exercise over and over and over again, like a game, regardless of pitch. So I thought to myself, "What if someone actually did 10,000 repetitions of any particular exercise such as a Siren? Would that allow them to perfect the exercise and strengthen their voice?" I knew the answer was "Yes" based on my Falsetto Siren days. In addition, I've been *PractiSing* myself and I've noticed an ease in my range stretching even before reaching 2,000 Lip Bubbles. How did I count that high? Did I use my fingers? Nope, I'm a little smarter than that. I downloaded a basic clicker app for my iPhone and then started doing Lip Bubbles throughout the day. Whenever I thought of it, I'd do one, two, or ten Lip Bubbles and click away on my clicker to keep a tally. I LOVE the 10,000 Challenge so much that I promise to add a clicker to TUNED XD in the near future, if it isn't already in there by the time you read this eBook.

So, the 10,000 Challenge will DEFINITELY drive you crazy mad about practice. You'll become obsessed, like 10,000 reps is your new drug. What exercise should you do? That is up to you. It can be a simple Lip Bubble slide down an octave and back up, or it could be one of my Isolation exercises, or even a vocal scale like the Miner Miner Mines from *Jim Gillette's Vocal Power*. If you do choose a vocal scale, please note that one rep equals one performance of the scale. In other words, if you typically start on the C below middle C and work up to Tenor C, that's a whole lot of reps. With the 10,000 Challenge, it isn't your typical scale work approach. You just do the scale pattern and that's it, one rep done, so click your clicker once. But our goal with the 10,000 Challenge is to push the limits of our range. So, whatever exercise you use, always attempt to start at the extreme high or low end, depending on whether you're working on your high range or low range.

Since I am working on my high range, each time I perform one rep of the 10,000 Challenge I try to start the Lip Bubble sound as high in pitch as possible without pushing it or straining it. For the first 500 or 600 I was probably reaching only a Tenor D or E, but then something weird happened. My voice blossomed and I was nailing Soprano B and C in the easiest, lightest voice imaginable, with crystal-clear tone. The 10,000 Challenge works!

Pssst— You can also use a pitch counter instead of a clicker app, which is a hand-held counter used in sports training. You can buy one at any sporting goods store. I tied a piece of nylon rope around its handle to make a necklace so I could hang my pitch counter around my neck for easy access.

THE PERCENTAGE DEDUCTION TECHNIQUE

PractiSing will overcome procrastination by changing your workout time to 5 a.m., first starting with the Mirror Mindset technique and then moving on to your vocal exercises, followed by working on your 10,000 Challenge throughout your day. But sometimes we have this little voice of doubt in the back of our minds, so we need an even quieter, calmer voice to reassure us we are doing the right thing, a little invisible pat on the back, a subconscious incentive to keep us marching forth. The Percentage Deduction Technique was another part of my dream, brought forth by my creative mindset. If the phrase "creative mindset" confuses you, check out my book *Unleash Your Creative Mindset*. You won't be disappointed, as it is the perfect companion to *PractiSing*, especially for those of you who write songs.

The Percentage Deduction Technique is a way to calculate how long you think you'll need to overcome any obstacle. I actually used this technique when I entered hypochondriac mode upon returning from a television show in Tokyo, Japan. I had caught some weird bug that affected the left side of my tongue, my left adenoid, left sinus passage, and left side of my epiglottis. I even lost my taste for several weeks. I tried various concoctions to overcome this weird illness, which aggravated the left-side lining of my throat without affecting my vocal cords. I did start to recover, but I think I was a bit scarred mentally, never having experienced something so drastic.

I immediately applied the Percentage Deduction Technique to my situation. In a notebook (actually on my iPhone) I wrote that each day I would become better by 4%. In my notes, once per day, I wrote:

4%
8%
12%
16%
And so on ...

I could feel myself reaching my goal. My pain was subsiding and whatever felt like it was stuck in my throat was shrinking. I know it's a simple subconscious trick, but it works, and it will help to instill the desire to overcome any obstacle you might be facing. An obstacle for you might be that you're having trouble performing Lip Bubbles, but you know that if you stay with it, you can overcome the problem in 20 days. Well, 20 days into 100 would be 5% per day. So, each day in your diary (or on your cell phone notepad or whatever works best for you), you'd put:

5%
10%
15%
And so on.

If you just cannot take your voice beyond the F above middle C, train hard and don't lose patience. Could you achieve that goal in 50 days? Do you truly believe you'll own that F in 50 days? Great, that means you'll be 2% closer every single day, so start a percentage list and go from 2%, 4%, 6%, 8%, etc., daily until you've reached 100%. I guarantee you'll reach your goal, as long as you're also *PractiSing*, and I'm betting you go beyond that F note!

One final note: If you happen to forget one day to write in the percentage, you CANNOT cheat and add it or skip over it. You've lost that percentage growth for one day and will have to continue with a day lost. Your 50-day process will take 51 days to complete. Don't let it discourage you; it's fine if it happens. In fact, it happened to me after I reached 20%. I forgot to write 24% the next day, so the following day I wrote 24% and picked up where I left off. There is nothing metaphysical about this; this is simply a subconscious megaphone screaming at your brain to help you achieve your goal.

And that is *PractiSing* in a nutshell. It WILL work, BUT you have to apply what I've laid out for you. It doesn't matter if you're using my exercises or any other exercise from any other vocal coach, the process is the same. Start early in the morning at 5 a.m. and accept the 10,000 Challenge. If you need a boost, apply the Percentage Deduction Technique. Now, on to my final thought ...

FINAL THOUGHT

I love adding final thoughts. I do it in many of my books and in each session of the Vendera Vocal Academy. So, this is *PractiSing* in a nutshell:

1—Address any excuse for not practicing, change the sentence, and repeat the new sentence every morning to yourself in the mirror at 5 a.m.
2—Self-evaluate your voice once per week.
3—Write out your vocal success goal map.

4—Start your vocal exercises at 5 a.m. after your mirror time. This also includes anything such as the Mindset program, breathing exercises, and cardio, as all your mind/body work is best done in the morning.
5—Keep a Vocal Workout Journal every day.
6—Accept a 10,000 Challenge and stick to it.
7—Use the Percentage Deduction Technique to overcome any obstacles.

That's it, not difficult at all! Now, get to *PractiSing* and I'll see you next book. For all my fans, you KNOW my next book isn't too far around the corner.

C-ya.

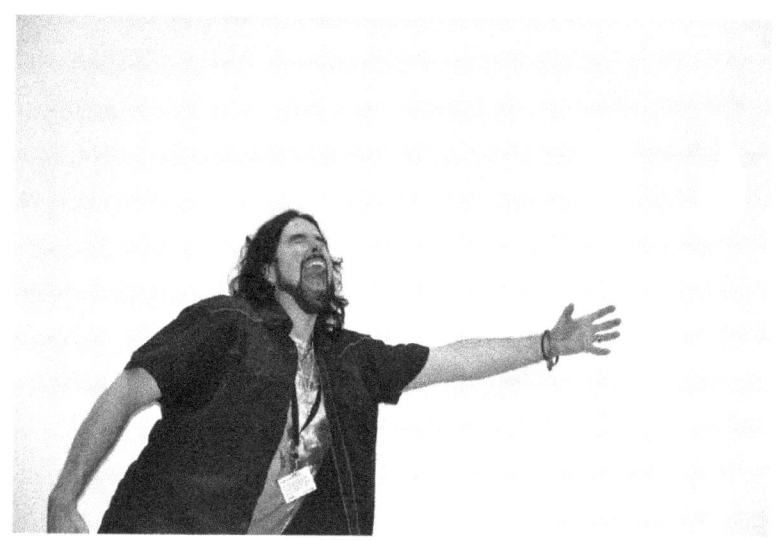

Jaime Vendera is the author of a variety books and one of the most sought-after vocal coaches on the planet. Using the methods that he created, Jaime turned his two-octave range into six octaves with massive decibels of raw vocal power that enabled him to set a world record, shattering glass with his voice. When singers need more vocal range, power, and projection, or need to build up vocal stamina to perform every night, they call Jaime Vendera. Jaime states that "none of this would have been possible without God."

    Ben Thomas of Dweezil Zappa says that Jaime is the "Mr. Miyagi" of vocal coaches, while Mat Devine of Kill Hannah considers him more of a "Yoda." James LaBrie of Dream Theater said, "Because of my lessons with Jaime, my voice is feeling and sounding better than it has in twenty years. I am spot-on every night. He is the Vocal Guru." Myles Kennedy of Alter Bridge said, "One time during a tour, I was so sick I could barely make it through the set. It looked as if we were going to have to cancel the next show. Jaime spent some time giving me some tips that helped me regain my voice. By the next night, I was able to perform the show. He is fantastic! Raise Your Voice Second Edition is THE book for singers. I recommend his books and his private instruction to ALL singers." Jaime can be contacted at jaimevendera.com.

www.ingramcontent.com/pod-product-compliance
Lightning Source LLC
Chambersburg PA
CBHW062119080426
42734CB00012B/2916